Airway Management UPDATES

Fast-Track Updates for Busy Clinicians

2025 EDITION

Authors

Prof. D. John Doyle, MD, PhD

Prof. Admir Hadzic, MD, PhD

NYSORA® PRESS

Publishing Division of NYSORA, Inc

2585 Broadway, suite 183, New York, NY10025

info@nysora.com, www.nysora.com

Contributors

- Dr. Imran Ahmad, MD, FRCA | Department of Anesthesiology and Critical care, Guy's & St Thomas' NHS Foundation Trust, London, UK
- Stien Beyens, MSc | NYSORA, Leuven, Belgium
- Prof. Tim Cook, FRCA, FICM | Professor of Anesthesiology, School of Medicine, University of Bristol, Bristol, UK
- Jirka Cops, PhD | NYSORA, Leuven, Belgium
- Prof. Ehab Farag, MD, FRCA,FASA | Professor of Anesthesiology, Cleveland Clinic Lerner College of Medicine, Case Western University, Cleveland, Ohio, USA | Department of Anesthesiology, Cleveland Clinic, Cleveland, Ohio, USA
- Prof. Carin Hagberg, MD, FASA | Professor of Anesthesiology, Department of Anesthesiology and Perioperative Medicine, University of Texas MD Anderson Center, Houston, Texas, USA
- Prof. Safaa Hilal, MD | Professor of Anesthesiology, Department of ICU and Pain Management, Menoufia university, Shibin Al Kawm, Al Minufiyah, Egypt
- Darren Jacobs, MSc | NYSORA, Leuven, Belgium
- Prof. Narasimhan 'Sim' Jagannathan, MD,MBA | Professor of Anesthesiology, College of Medicine, University of Arizona, Phoenix, Arizona, USA | Department of Anesthesiology, Phoenix Children's, Phoenix, Arizona, USA
- Dr. Fadi Kadourra, MD | Department of Anesthesia and Pain Medicine, Sheikh Shakhbout Medical City (SSMC), Abu Dhabi, Unites Arab Emirates
- Dr. Daniel Perin, MD, PhD | Department of Anesthesiology, Hospital Albert Einstein, São Paulo, Brazil
- Prof. William Rosenblatt, MD | Professor of Anesthesiology, Department of Anesthesiology, Yale University School of Medicine, New Haven, Connecticut, USA
- Dr. Mona Sarkiss, MD, PhD | Department of Anesthesiology and Perioperative Medicine and Department of Pulmonary Medicine, University of Texas MD Anderson Center, Houston, Texas, USA
- Prof. Peter Slinger, MD, FRCPC | Professor of Anesthesiology, Department of Anesthesiology and Pain Medicine, University of Toronto, Toronto, Canada
- Jill Vanhaeren, MSc | NYSORA, Leuven, Belgium
- Dr. Yasser Zaghloul, MD | Anesthesiology institute, Sheikh Khalifa Medical City, Abu Dhabi, United Arab Emirates

Introduction

Every year, the world of medicine evolves, bringing forth groundbreaking research, clinical guidelines, and innovative techniques that shape the way we manage airway challenges. However, the sheer volume of information-spread across journals, conferences, and online platforms-can feel overwhelming and fragmented. While social media and informal channels offer glimpses of these advancements, they often lack the depth and reliability essential for sound clinical decisions.

Airway Management Updates 2025 was created to bridge this gap, providing you with a trusted, streamlined resource for the most significant developments in airway management from the past couple of years. NYSORA's editorial team has meticulously curated and distilled these advancements into concise, easy-to-read updates that can be absorbed in just 10 minutes.

To ensure the highest quality and relevance, each topic underwent our **Internal Peer-Review Process**, followed by **External Peer Review** by NYSORA's International Editorial Board. This board includes a balanced mix of top experts, researchers, educators, and practicing clinicians who contributed to building a consensus on what matters most for clinical practice in 2025.

This edition contains **48 concise and engaging updates**, reflecting the most critical findings from clinical trials, consensus recommendations, industry developments, and guidelines over the past 3 years. Each update is designed to refresh your knowledge and offer actionable insights that can be immediately applied to patient care. The content is organized into clearly defined sections for easy navigation, with ample space for your personal notes to customize the material for your unique needs.

To simplify further exploration, we've included only key references for those seeking more in-depth information on a given topic.

Our hope is that **Airway Management Updates 2025** will serve as your go-to resource, helping you stay ahead in the rapidly evolving field of airway management. With this book, we aim to empower clinicians to optimize patient care through knowledge that is both practical and cutting-edge.

Dedication

To the clinicians who strive every day to improve the lives of their patients and to the educators and researchers whose dedication to advancing the field makes this possible-this book is for you.

Your commitment to excellence inspires progress, and it is our privilege to support your journey. May Airway Management Updates 2025 serve as a trusted companion in your pursuit of knowledge, growth, and the highest standards of care.

Acknowledgements

I would like to express my deepest gratitude to my clinical colleagues around the world who have tirelessly advanced the field of clinical airway management, year after year, through their dedication, innovation, and unwavering commitment to patient care. Their collective expertise and contributions have continually elevated both the efficacy and safety of airway interventions, shaping the standards and best practices that benefit patients globally.

A special note of appreciation goes to NYSORA's editorial team for their invaluable support, keen insights, and unwavering encouragement, which have played a pivotal role in bringing this project to life. Their dedication and assistance have been instrumental in refining and realizing this endeavor, and for that, I am truly grateful.

Finally, I would like to acknowledge NYSORA's talented staff of designers and desktop publishers. Your creativity and attention to detail have transformed this content into a reader-friendly format, making the material accessible and easy to navigate for all readers.

With deep appreciation,
Prof. Dr. D. John Doyle, MD, PhD

Notice / Disclaimer

Errata: While every effort has been made to ensure the accuracy and quality of this book, errors or areas for improvement may still exist. If you identify any inaccuracies or have suggestions for enhancing the content or visuals, please send your feedback to info@nysora.com. We value your input and may acknowledge contributions as appropriate. Thank you for supporting our commitment to continuous improvement.

Library of Congress Identification

Authors: **John Doyle, MD, PhD | Admir Hadzic, MD, PhD**

Title: Airway Management Updates
Subtitle: Fast-Track Updates for Busy Clinicians
2025 Edition

Identifiers:
Library of Congress Control Number: 2025900054
ISBN: 978-1-966637-00-4

Table of Contents

Specialized airway management techniques

Education and technology in airway management

Airway safety and risk management

Miscellaneous

General guidelines and recommendations

Guidelines for awake intubation from the Difficult Airway Society

01

Why this topic is important

Awake tracheal intubation (ATI) is vital in managing predicted difficult airways. It allows clinicians to secure the airway while preserving the patient's spontaneous breathing and airway reflexes. This reduces the risks associated with failed intubation during general anesthesia, such as hypoxia or airway trauma. Despite its safety and efficacy, ATI still needs to be utilized, with reports showing it is performed in only 0.2% of tracheal intubations in the UK.

Barriers to wider adoption include lack of familiarity, perceived complexity, and concerns about patient comfort. The updated Difficult Airway Society (DAS) guidelines aim to address these challenges. By standardizing preparation, performance, and management strategies, the guidelines seek to lower the threshold for using ATI, improving its accessibility and safety for clinicians across varying levels of experience.

Objectives of this update

- To provide a structured framework for safe and effective ATI.
- To outline best practices for sedation, topicalization, oxygenation, and performance (sTOP).
- To highlight strategies for complication management and escalation protocols.

What is new

The DAS guidelines introduce a systematic approach to ATI, incorporating key updates:

- STOP framework: A focus on Sedation, Topicalization, Oxygenation, and Performance.
- Checklists and cognitive aids: Emphasized for preparation and intra-procedure efficiency.
- Clear escalation protocols: Defined for managing failed ATI attempts, including limits on intubation attempts and strategies for transitioning to alternative techniques.

Indications for awake tracheal intubation

- ATI should be considered in patients with predictors of difficult airway management, such as:
- Reduced neck mobility or mouth opening.
- Airway obstruction due to masses, trauma, or infection.
- Obesity, obstructive sleep apnea, or prior difficult airway history.

Poor patient cooperation, active airway bleeding, or local anesthetic allergies are relative contraindications. Patient refusal is an absolute contraindication.

Preparation and procedural setup

1. **Environment:**
   - Perform ATI in a fully equipped operating room with immediate access to emergency airway devices.
   - The same care standards apply in critical scenarios, such as ICU or emergency settings.
2. **Team readiness:**
   - Assign specific roles to team members. Use cognitive aids, such as checklists, to ensure preparation completeness.
3. **Patient positioning:**
   - Position the patient semi-upright to optimize airway access and oxygenation.

Sedation and topicalization

1. **Sedation:**
   - Minimal sedation is preferred, sufficient to reduce anxiety without compromising spontaneous ventilation.
   - Remifentanil and dexmedetomidine are recommended agents due to their safety profiles.
   - Avoid propofol as a sole sedative, given its higher risk of oversedation.
2. **Topicalization:**
   - Lidocaine (up to 9 mg/kg lean body weight) can be used for local anesthesia of the airway structures.
   - Apply through sprays, nebulization, or atomizers, ensuring thorough coverage before proceeding.

Oxygenation

- Administer supplemental oxygen throughout the procedure, ideally using high-flow nasal oxygen (HFNO).
- Monitor oxygen saturation continuously, ensuring desaturation events are promptly addressed.

Performance of ATI

1. **Technique selection:**
   - Flexible bronchoscopy (FB) and video-laryngoscopy (VL) are the primary tools, with comparable success rates (~98%).
   - The choice of technique depends on the patient's anatomy and operator experience.
2. **Confirmation of tube placement:**
   - Perform a two-point check: direct visualization of the trachea and confirmation with capnography.

3. **Attempts:**
    - Limit intubation attempts to three, with one additional attempt by a senior clinician if necessary.

Management of failed ATI

1. **Escalation strategy:**
    - Reassess and optimize sedation, topica-lization, or technique after each failed attempt.
    - Transition to alternative airway strategies if ATI remains unsuccessful, including supraglottic devices or front-of-neck access (FONA).
2. **Team communication:**
    - Communicate the need for escalation, ensuring all team members are aligned on the next steps.

Training and competency

- Training should include simulation and supervised clinical practice, focusing on technical and non-technical skills.
- Institutions should provide regular opportunities for skill maintenance and reinforce the use of cognitive aids.

Clinical implications

The DAS guidelines provide a comprehensive framework for ATI, emphasizing preparation, systematic execution, and structured escalation. This approach reduces risks and enhances procedural efficiency and patient outcomes. By making ATI more accessible and standardized, the guidelines aim to increase its utilization in patients at high risk for airway difficulties.

These recommendations also address patient-centered care, emphasizing comfort, communication, and tailored management to ensure a positive experience.

Key takeaways

☑ ATI is a safe and effective technique for securing difficult airways while preserving patient spontaneous ventilation.

☑ Preparation, including minimal sedation and effective topicalization, is critical for success.

☑ The sTOP framework offers a systematic approach to ATI, improving safety and efficiency.

☑ Escalate to alternative airway strategies after three failed attempts, emphasizing structured decision-making.

☑ Regular training and the use of cognitive aids are essential to maintain competency and improve outcomes.

Additional recommended reading:

1. Ahmad I, El-Boghdadly K, Bhagrath R, et al. Difficult Airway Society guidelines for awake tracheal intubation in adults. *Anaesthesia*. 2020;75(4):509-528. PMID: 31729018; PMCID: PMC7078877.
2. Frerk C, Mitchell VS, McNarry AF, et al. Difficult Airway Society 2015 guidelines for management of unanticipated difficult intubation in adults. *Br J Anaesth*. 2015;115:827-848. PMID: 26556848; PMCID: PMC4650961.
3. Cook TM, MacDougall-Davis SR. Complications and failure of airway management. *Br J Anaesth*. 2012;109:68-85. PMID: 23242753.

ASA guidelines for managing difficult airways

02

Why this topic is important

Managing difficult airways is one of the most critical responsibilities for anesthesiologists and other healthcare professionals involved in airway management. The failure to secure an airway promptly can lead to catastrophic complications, including hypoxia, brain injury, cardiac arrest, and death. Difficult airway scenarios-whether anticipated or unanticipated-demand meticulous preparation, skillful execution, and an adaptive approach.

The American Society of Anesthesiologists (ASA) 2022 guidelines for managing the difficult airway incorporate significant updates. They address the challenges of technological advancements, evolving clinical practices, and patient-specific factors such as obesity and craniofacial abnormalities. These guidelines emphasize a standardized yet flexible approach, offering new tools, refined algorithms, and evidence-based recommendations to improve outcomes.

The importance of these updates cannot be overstated. In clinical practice, anesthesiologists and other clinicians frequently face high-pressure situations requiring quick decision-making. The 2022 guidelines provide a framework for anticipating airway difficulties, preparing appropriate equipment and strategies, and executing interventions safely and effectively.

Objectives of this update

- Highlight key updates to the ASA guidelines for managing difficult airways.
- Provide insights into new recommendations for airway assessment, equipment preparation, and advanced techniques.
- Offer actionable routine and emergency airway management strategies in pediatric and adult patients.

What is new

The 2022 ASA guidelines introduce significant revisions and additions compared to the 2012 version, reflecting new evidence and clinical priorities:

- Focus on continuous oxygenation: Emphasis on administering supplemental oxygen throughout airway management, including during extubation, to prevent hypoxia.
- Updated algorithms: Revised and simplified decision-making pathways tailored to adult and pediatric patients.
- Limited intubation attempts: It is strongly recommended that the number of intubation attempts be restricted to reduce airway trauma and complications.
- Refined extubation strategies: Guidelines on extubation in patients with difficult airways, including staged extubation techniques and airway exchange catheters.
- Incorporation of new tools: Integration of advanced airway devices such as video laryngoscopes, supraglottic airway (SGA) devices, and emergency cricothyrotomy kits.

Key findings

Comprehensive airway evaluation

- Risk assessment:
  - If necessary, conduct a detailed preoperative evaluation using patient history, physical examination, and diagnostic imaging.
  - Traditional predictors such as Mallampati classification, thyromental distance, and neck mobility are combined with advanced modalities like airway ultrasound to improve diagnostic accuracy.
- Structured planning:
  - Categorize the airway as normal, anticipated difficult, or unanticipated difficult.
  - Develop a stepwise management plan, considering alternative techniques and backup strategies.

Equipment and preparation

- Standardized airway cart:
  - Ensure the availability of essential devices, including bag-mask ventilation (BMV), direct laryngoscopes, video laryngoscopes, bougies, SGAs, and cricothyrotomy kits.
- Supplemental oxygenation:
  - Use a high-flow nasal cannula (HFNC) or similar devices to maintain oxygenation during apneic periods.
  - Continue oxygen delivery throughout preoxygenation, intubation, and extubation.
- Advanced devices:
  - Familiarize the team with airway evaluation and management tools, such as flexible bronchoscopes, rigid intubation scopes, and ultrasound.

Strategies for anticipated difficult airways

- Awake intubation:
  - Perform awake intubation in cases with predicted difficulty in both intubation and ventilation.
  - Use flexible bronchoscopic guidance or videolaryngoscopy to prioritize patient comfort and safety.
- Sequential device use:
  - Predefine a stepwise sequence for attempting devices, minimizing the number of attempts to prevent trauma.
  - Transition to alternative techniques like SGA or cricothyrotomy if intubation fails.

Management of unanticipated difficult airways

- Calling for help:
  - Activate the difficult airway response team immediately upon recognizing airway challenges.
  - Ensure all personnel are aware of their roles and responsibilities.
- Noninvasive approaches:
  - Begin with BMV to maintain oxygenation, and transition to SGAs if ventilation is difficult.
- Emergency invasive techniques:
  - Be prepared to perform cricothyrotomy or other invasive procedures when noninvasive methods fail.

Extubation strategies

- Extubation in difficult airway patients:
  - Use airway exchange catheters or staged extubation plans for high-risk patients.
  - Ensure the immediate availability of re-intubation equipment and expertise.
- Supplemental oxygen post-extubation:
  - Continue oxygen therapy post-extubation to mitigate hypoxia, especially in patients with residual airway edema or other risk factors.

Clinical implications

Improving outcomes through structured preparation

These guidelines reinforce the importance of preemptive planning and team coordination in airway management. Structured preparation, including comprehensive risk assessment and appropriate equipment readiness, minimizes complications and improves the likelihood of successful airway management.

Integrating advanced tools and techniques

Incorporating videolaryngoscopy, airway ultrasound, and cognitive aids underscores the evolving landscape of airway management. Familiarity with these tools is essential for ensuring safety and efficiency in clinical practice.

Enhancing patient safety

Recommendations to limit intubation attempts and adopt continuous oxygenation strategies directly address common complications like airway trauma and hypoxia. These updates prioritize patient safety while maintaining clinical effectiveness.

Limitations

- Real-world applications may vary due to resource availability, especially in low-resource settings.
- Adopting newer technologies requires training and proficiency, which may limit immediate implementation.

Key takeaways

- ☑ Conduct thorough airway evaluations using a combination of physical examination, history, and advanced diagnostic tools.
- ☑ Maintain supplemental oxygen throughout all phases of airway management to prevent hypoxia.
- ☑ Restrict intubation attempts and adopt sequential device strategies to minimize complications.
- ☑ Prepare for extubation in difficult airway patients with staged approaches and reintubation readiness.
- ☑ Familiarize the team with advanced tools like video laryngoscopes and cognitive aids to enhance success rates.

Additional recommended reading:

1. Apfelbaum JL, Hagberg CA, Connis RT, et al. 2022 American Society of Anesthesiologists practice guidelines for management of the difficult airway. *Anesthesiology*. 2022;136(1):31-81. PMID: 34762729.
2. Cook TM, MacDougall-Davis SR. Complications and failure of airway management. *Br J Anaesth*. 2012;109(1):68-85. PMID: 23242753.
3. Altun D, Kara H, Bozbora E, et al. The Role of Indirect Laryngoscopy, Clinical and Ultrasonographic Assessment in Prediction of Difficult Airway. Laryngoscope. 2021;131(2):E555-E560. PMID: 32730647.

European airway management guideline for neonates and infants

03

Why this topic is important

Airway management in neonates and infants is a cornerstone of safe and effective anesthesia care. These youngest patients are particularly vulnerable due to their unique anatomy, immature physiology, and small airway size, which increase the risks of hypoxemia, airway trauma, and rapid deterioration during procedures. The complexity of managing their airways necessitates clear, evidence-based guidelines to standardize care and minimize complications.

Recognizing the challenges of neonatal and infant airway management, the European Society of Anaesthesiology and Intensive Care (ESAIC), in collaboration with the British Journal of Anaesthesia (BJA), published a comprehensive guideline. This update integrates the latest evidence and expert consensus, addressing all critical aspects of airway management, from preoperative assessment to post-extubation care, with a focus on safety and effectiveness.

Objectives of this update

- Summarize key recommendations from the European airway management guideline for neonates and infants.
- Discuss practical implications for clinicians, including preoperative preparation, intubation techniques, and post-extubation strategies.
- Highlight the importance of interdisciplinary collaboration and ongoing education in improving airway management outcomes.

What is new

The guideline introduces ten key recommendations informed by a structured review of recent literature and a three-step Delphi consensus process. Key highlights include:

- Videolaryngoscopy (VL) is the first-line device for tracheal intubation in neonates and infants.
- Use of neuromuscular blocking agents (NMBAs) to optimize intubation conditions.
- Adoption of apnoeic oxygenation and post-extubation respiratory support techniques, such as high-flow nasal oxygen (HFNO) and continuous positive airway pressure (CPAP), to reduce complications.

Key recommendations for neonatal and infant airway management

1. **Preoperative assessment and preparation**

- **Medical history and physical examination:**
  - Assess for congenital abnormalities, craniofacial syndromes, and other risk factors for difficult airways.
  - Use this information to anticipate challenges and prepare alternative strategies, including rescue techniques.
- **Team readiness:**
  - Ensure an experienced team with defined roles is available, especially for high-risk cases.

2. **Neuromuscular blocking agents**

- Administer NMBAs unless spontaneous breathing is required to maintain oxygenation (e.g., in specific cases of congenital diaphragmatic hernia).
- NMBAs improve intubation conditions and reduce airway trauma by relaxing the vocal cords and preventing patient movement.

3. **Videolaryngoscopy as the first choice**

- VL is recommended over direct laryngoscopy (DL) due to its superior visualization and higher first-pass success rates.
- Use hyperangulated blades and stylets for anteriorly positioned larynxes or challenging airways.

4. **Apnoeic oxygenation**

- Provide oxygenation during laryngoscopy using HFNO or low-flow nasal oxygen to prolong safe apnea time.
- Apnoeic oxygenation is particularly important in neonates, who desaturate rapidly due to their high oxygen consumption and small functional residual capacity.

Why videolaryngoscopy (VL) matters in neonates
Improves success rates in small, anterior airways.
Reduces the need for repeated attempts, minimizing trauma.
Allows team members to view intubation in real time, improving communication.

5. **Rescue techniques**

- If intubation fails:
  - Use supraglottic airway devices (SGAs) as a bridge to ventilation.
  - Minimize repeated intubation attempts to reduce trauma and complications.
- Ensure the availability of advanced airway tools, such as flexible bronchoscopes.

6. Postextubation respiratory support

- Use HFNO, CPAP, or nasal positive pressure ventilation (NPPV) to prevent post-extubation atelectasis and respiratory failure.
- Tailor respiratory support to the patient's condition, adjusting parameters based on lung compliance and oxygenation needs.

7. Confirmation of tracheal intubation

- Verify tube placement using capnography and bilateral chest auscultation.
- Use videolaryngoscopy or ultrasonography as adjuncts in cases of uncertainty.

Airway management workflow for neonates and infants	
1. Preoperative assessment	History → Physical exam → Risk stratification
2. Intubation steps	• Use of VL as first-line • Administration of NMBAs • Apnoeic oxygenation strategies
3. Confirmation of tube placement	• Capnography • Auscultation • Ultrasound (if needed)
4. Rescue techniques	SGAs → Flexible bronchoscopy → Advanced airway tools
5. Post-extubation care	HFNO, CPAP, and NPPV

Interdisciplinary collaboration and education

- The guideline emphasizes the importance of a cohesive, interdisciplinary team approach, with clear role allocation and communication strategies such as closed-loop feedback.
- Simulation-based training is highlighted as essential for developing and maintaining airway management skills, particularly in low-caseload centers.

Limitations

The guideline acknowledges gaps in evidence for certain recommendations:

1. **Limited studies in neonates:**
   - Many studies included in the review were conducted in older children or simulated environments.
   - Neonate-specific trials are needed to validate findings and refine protocols.
2. **Emerging techniques:**
   - Novel approaches, such as less invasive surfactant administration (LISA), were not covered comprehensively and warrant further research.

Practical implications for clinicians

Preparation and readiness

- Develop standardized airway management protocols aligned with the guidelines to ensure consistency in care.
- Integrate VL and advanced airway tools into routine practice, with training sessions focused on their use.

Individualizing care

- Tailor interventions based on the patient's anatomy, underlying conditions, and procedure requirements.
- Implement apnoeic oxygenation and post-extubation support strategies to reduce complications.

Fostering teamwork and education

- Encourage regular team-based training sessions, including simulations of difficult airway scenarios.
- Invest in ongoing education to stay updated on advancements in neonatal and infant airway management.

Key takeaways

☑ Neonates and infants present unique airway management challenges requiring specialized skills, preparation, and equipment.

☑ Videolaryngoscopy should be the first-line device for tracheal intubation, improving visualization and success rates.

☑ Neuromuscular blocking agents and apnoeic oxygenation enhance safety and reduce complications during intubation.

☑ Post-extubation respiratory support, such as HFNO and CPAP, is essential for preventing respiratory failure.

☑ Interdisciplinary collaboration and structured education programs are vital to improving neonatal airway management outcomes.

<u>**Additional recommended reading:**</u>

1. Hansen TG, Aunsholt L, Weiss M. Ensuring the brightest start: the new European airway management guideline for neonates and infants. *Eur J Anaesthesiol.* 2024;41(1):1-2. PMID: 38054216.
2. Disma N, Asai T, Cools E, et al. Airway management in neonates and infants: European Society of Anaesthesiology and Intensive Care and British Journal of Anaesthesia joint guidelines. *Eur J Anaesthesiol.* 2024;41(3-23). PMID: 38018248; PMCID: PMC10720842.
3. Sweet DG, Carnielli VC, Greisen G, et al. European consensus guidelines on the management of respiratory distress syndrome: 2022 update. *Neonatology*. 2023;120:3-23. PMID: 36863329; PMCID: PMC10064400.

The 2022 ASA difficult airway algorithm decision tree approach

04

Why this topic is important

Effective airway management is a cornerstone of anesthetic practice. Failure to secure the airway can lead to catastrophic outcomes such as hypoxia, aspiration, and cardiac arrest. Recognizing and preparing for difficult airways is vital for reducing complications and ensuring patient safety.

The American Society of Anesthesiologists (ASA) first introduced the Difficult Airway Algorithm in 1993 to provide structured guidance in airway management. However, earlier versions lacked specificity in decision-making pathways, particularly in choosing between awake intubation and general anesthesia induction. The 2022 revision introduces a decision tree framework, integrating key patient factors and clinical contexts to improve decision-making precision and adaptability. This new tool aims to enhance communication, promote systematic assessment, and reduce the risks associated with airway management failures.

Objectives of this update

- Explain the role and structure of the 2022 ASA Difficult Airway Algorithm decision tree.
- Highlight critical decision-making elements, including risk assessments for intubation, ventilation, aspiration, and apnea tolerance.
- Recommend integrating the decision tree approach into clinical practice to optimize patient outcomes.

What is new

- A decision tree tool is introduced to guide choices between awake intubation and airway management post-general anesthesia induction.
- Emphasis on inductive assessments considering patient anatomy, aspiration risks, desaturation potential, and clinical context.
- Integration of individualized assessments of anesthesiologists' skills, resources, and patient cooperation into the decision-making process.

Key findings

The four key elements of airway decision-making

1. Risk of difficult laryngoscopy and tracheal intubation:
    - While bedside airway assessments, such as Mallampati scoring, remain standard, their predictive accuracy is limited.
    - The decision tree advocates combining anatomical assessments with the anesthesiologist's expertise and patient-specific factors to estimate intubation success.
2. Facemask or supraglottic ventilation feasibility:
    - If facemask or supraglottic airway ventilation is deemed nonviable, the likelihood of a "cannot-intubate, cannot-ventilate" (CICV) scenario increases, favoring the awake intubation pathway.
3. Aspiration risk:
    - Significant aspiration risks necessitate careful consideration of awake intubation to secure the airway without inducing apnea.
4. Tolerance for apnea:
    - Patients with compromised physiologies, such as obesity, pregnancy, or severe hypoxemia, may not tolerate even brief apnea, pushing the decision toward awake intubation.

Awake intubation as a safe pathway

- Awake intubation is considered the safest approach for patients predicted to have difficult airways or CICV scenarios.
- While effective, it requires skilled execution and may be influenced by patient cooperation and sedation-related risks.

The role of contextual and operator factors

- Decisions are not one-size-fits-all but reflect the anesthesiologist's expertise, available resources, and the case's urgency.
- Collaboration with experienced colleagues or specialists is encouraged when challenges exceed the primary anesthesiologist's skill set.

Recommendations for practice

Decision-making and preparation

1. Incorporate the decision tree framework:
    - Use the tool to systematically assess key factors, including intubation and ventilation difficulty, aspiration risk, and apnea tolerance.
2. Prepare for awake intubation:
    - Develop proficiency in awake techniques through simulation training and incorporate tools like flexible bronchoscopes and videolaryngoscopy into routine practice.
3. Anticipate rescue scenarios:
    - Establish a backup plan for CICV situations, including supraglottic airway devices and invasive airway techniques (e.g., cricothyrotomy).

Enhancing skills and communication

- Ongoing training: Regularly participate in workshops and simulations to improve decision-making confidence and technical skills for awake and post-induction intubations.
- Interdisciplinary collaboration: Involve surgeons and critical care teams early when managing patients with high airway risks.

Practical implementation

- Adapt plans based on patient-specific needs: Adjust airway strategies for individual patients, particularly those with unique anatomical or physiological challenges.
- Leverage resources and expertise: Recognize when external assistance is required and ensure appropriate equipment and personnel are available.

Broader implications

The 2022 ASA Difficult Airway Algorithm's decision tree represents a significant advance in airway management. It offers a systematic approach to navigating complex clinical scenarios. By prioritizing patient safety and tailoring strategies to individual circumstances, the tool facilitates better communication, reduces complications, and enhances emergency preparedness.

Future directions include:

- Developing objective risk assessment tools to complement the decision tree and improve predictive accuracy.
- Expanding education and accessibility of awake intubation techniques to support widespread adoption.
- Evaluating the decision tree's impact on clinical outcomes through multicenter studies.

Key takeaways

☑ The 2022 ASA Difficult Airway Algorithm introduces a decision tree tool to guide airway management, emphasizing risk assessments for intubation, ventilation, aspiration, and apnea.

☑ Awake intubation is preferred for high-risk patients, particularly those with anticipated CICV scenarios or reduced apnea tolerance.

☑ Decisions must consider patient factors, clinical context, and the anesthesiologist's expertise, promoting individualized and adaptive care.

☑ Ongoing training and interdisciplinary collaboration are essential for maximizing the tool's utility and improving airway safety.

Additional recommended reading:

1. Rosenblatt WH, Yanez ND. A decision tree approach to airway management pathways in the 2022 Difficult Airway Algorithm of the American Society of Anesthesiologists. *Anesth Analg.* 2022;134(5):910-915. PMID: 35171880; PMCID: PMC8986631.
2. Apfelbaum JL, Hagberg CA, Caplan RA, et al. Practice guidelines for management of the difficult airway: an updated report by the ASA Task Force on Management of the Difficult Airway. *Anesthesiology*. 2022;136(1):31-50. PMID: 23364566.
3. Ahmad I, El-Boghdadly K, Bhagrath R, et al. Difficult Airway Society guidelines for awake tracheal intubation in adults. *Anaesthesia.* 2020;75(4):509—528. PMID: 31729018; PMCID: PMC7078877.

Consensus recommendations for the difficult airway

05

Why this topic is important

The physiologically difficult airway (PDA) represents a critical challenge in airway management, particularly in critically ill patients. Unlike anatomically difficult airways, PDAs involve physiological derangements such as hypoxemia, hypotension, or acidosis that complicate tracheal intubation and increase the risk of adverse events, including peri-intubation cardiac arrest and death. These complications highlight the need for a systematic, physiologically focused approach to airway management.

The Society for Airway Management (SAM) identified a gap in international guidelines addressing PDAs and convened a multidisciplinary team to develop evidence-based recommendations. These recommendations provide practical strategies to mitigate risks associated with intubating physiologically compromised patients. By emphasizing proactive management, SAM's guidelines aim to reduce the high morbidity and mortality linked to these scenarios while standardizing care across diverse settings.

Objectives of this update

- Explain the defining characteristics and challenges of managing PDAs in critically ill patients.
- Highlight consensus recommendations from SAM on preoxygenation, hemodynamic optimization, and managing high-risk physiological states.
- Discuss practical applications of these recommendations in diverse clinical settings to enhance patient outcomes.

What is new

- Detailed algorithms to guide preoxygenation strategies, including high-flow nasal oxygen (HFNO) and noninvasive positive pressure ventilation (NIPPV).
- Emphasis on mitigating hemodynamic instability with proactive fluid resuscitation and vasopressor support.
- Novel recommendations for managing specific high-risk scenarios, such as refractory hypoxemia, right ventricular dysfunction, and severe metabolic acidosis.

Key findings

Preoxygenation and apneic oxygenation

1. Optimizing oxygenation:
   - Preoxygenation with 100% oxygen for at least three minutes or eight vital capacity breaths is essential to delay desaturation during intubation.
   - HFNO is recommended for patients unable to maintain adequate oxygen saturation (> 93%) with a non-rebreather mask.
2. Apneic oxygenation:
   - During laryngoscopy, continuous oxygen delivery through nasal cannulas at 15 liters per minute (LPM) or HFNO prolongs the safe apnea time.
   - Patients with shunt physiology, such as those with acute respiratory distress syndrome (ARDS), require strategies to improve ventilation-perfusion (V/Q) mismatch, such as positive end-expiratory pressure (PEEP).

Hemodynamic stabilization

1. Identifying risk:
   - Patients with a shock index > 0.7 or pre-intubation hypotension are at high risk for hemodynamic collapse.
   - Preemptive fluid resuscitation is crucial in fluid-tolerant patients to maintain perfusion during intubation.
2. Vasopressor use:
   - Early initiation of norepinephrine infusions is recommended for patients at risk of or experiencing hypotension.
   - When continuous infusions are unavailable, bolus doses of epinephrine or phenylephrine can stabilize hemodynamics during induction.

Management of specific physiological challenges

1. Refractory hypoxemia:
   - In extreme cases, recruitment maneuvers, pulmonary vasodilators, and awake intubation are used to optimize oxygenation.
2. Right ventricular (RV) dysfunction:
   - Minimize RV afterload with pulmonary vasodilators and avoid excessive fluid resuscitation.
   - Preoxygenation strategies should prevent worsening V/Q mismatch and hypoxemia.
3. Severe metabolic acidosis:
   - High-minute ventilation requires awake or supported intubation techniques to avoid rapid respiratory decompensation.

Recommendations for practice

Before intubation

1. Perform comprehensive physiological assess-ments to identify risk factors for hypoxemia, hypotension, and metabolic acidosis.
2. Optimize preoxygenation with HFNO or NIPPV for at least three minutes to achieve end-tidal oxygen levels above 90%.
3. Administer fluids or vasopressors to maintain mean arterial pressure (MAP) > 65 mmHg, reducing the risk of peri-intubation cardiac arrest.

During intubation

1. To extend safe apnea time, utilize apneic oxygenation with high-flow nasal cannulas or other delivery systems.
2. Select induction agents tailored to the patient's physiological state, such as etomidate for hemodynamic neutrality or ketamine for hypotension.

After intubation

1. Reassess oxygenation and hemodynamics immediately, addressing complications such as pneumothorax or worsening pulmonary edema.
2. Implement ventilatory strategies tailored to the underlying physiology, such as low tidal volumes and optimal PEEP for ARDS.

Broader implications

Managing PDAs demands a multidisciplinary, physiologically informed approach that anticipates and mitigates risks before, during, and after intubation. The SAM recommendations offer a structured framework applicable across clinical environments, from emergency departments to intensive care units. In addition to improving patient outcomes, these guidelines provide a foundation for standardizing training and workflows, ultimately fostering consistency and confidence among clinicians managing high-risk airways.

Future directions include:

- Expanding training programs to equip clinicians with the skills to implement these recommendations.
- Conducting large-scale studies to validate the effectiveness of physiologically focused airway management strategies.
- Refining algorithms to integrate emerging technologies and evidence.

Key takeaways

☑ Physiologically difficult airways pose unique challenges requiring tailored preoxygenation, hemodynamic stabilization, and ventilatory strategies to optimize safety and outcomes.

☑ Preoxygenation with HFNO or NIPPV and apneic oxygenation significantly reduce the risk of desaturation during intubation.

☑ Fluid resuscitation, vasopressors, and careful selection of induction agents are critical to mitigating peri-intubation hypotension and related complications.

☑ SAM recommendations emphasize a proactive, patient-centered approach to improve outcomes in high-risk intubations, advocating for widespread training and standardization.

Additional recommended reading:

1. Kornas RL, Owyang CG, Sakles JC, et al. Evaluation and management of the physiologically difficult airway: Consensus recommendations from Society for Airway Management. *Anesth Analg.* 2021;132(2):395-405. PMID: 33060492.

2. Mosier JM, Sakles JC, Whitmore SP, et al. The physiologically difficult airway: Winning the race between desaturation and intubation. *Br J Anaesth.* 2020;125:e1-e4. PMID: 31882262.

3. Jaber S, Jung B, Corne P, et al. An intervention to decrease complications related to endotracheal intubation in the ICU: A prospective multicenter study. *Intensive Care Med.* 2010;36:248-255. PMID: 19921148.

Airway management in pediatric patients and neonates

Prevention of atelectasis by continuous positive airway pressure in children

06

Why this topic is important

Atelectasis, or alveolar collapse, is a common complication during general anesthesia, affecting patients across all age groups. In children, it can occur immediately after induction of anesthesia and can persist into the postoperative period. Atelectasis impairs gas exchange by creating a shunt effect, which increases the risk of hypoxemia and postoperative pulmonary complications.

Continuous positive airway pressure (CPAP) offers a potential solution by maintaining lung expansion during anesthesia. While the benefits of CPAP in preventing atelectasis are well-established in adults, its application in pediatric populations remains underexplored. A randomized controlled study by Acosta et al. (2021) investigated the efficacy of CPAP in preventing perioperative atelectasis in children, providing critical insights into its potential for improving pediatric anesthesia outcomes.

Objectives of this update

- Explore the role of CPAP during anesthesia induction and emergence in reducing atelectasis in children.
- Highlight key findings on CPAP's impact on lung aeration and postoperative outcomes.
- Provide practical recommendations for implementing CPAP in pediatric anesthesia.

What is new

The study by Acosta et al. confirms the efficacy of CPAP in preventing atelectasis during anesthesia induction and emergence:

- CPAP during induction reduced atelectasis incidence from 95% (control group) to 52%.
- Postoperative residual atelectasis was significantly lower in the CPAP group (10%) compared to the control group (30%).
- CPAP improved lung aeration scores and reduced the need for intraoperative recruitment maneuvers.

These findings underscore CPAP's value as a preventive strategy, marking an important step in optimizing pediatric anesthesia care.

Understanding the impact of CPAP

Baseline challenges in pediatric anesthesia

Induction of anesthesia leads to atelectasis through mechanisms such as airway closure, loss of diaphragmatic tone, and high inspired oxygen concentrations. These effects are more pronounced in children due to:

- **Smaller functional residual capacity (FRC):** Reduced lung reserves make children more vulnerable to alveolar collapse.
- **High oxygen consumption:** Rapid desaturation occurs during apnea, exacerbating hypoxemia.
- **Respiratory mechanics:** A compliant chest wall and immature lung architecture increase susceptibility to atelectasis.

Effects of CPAP during induction

1. **Reduced atelectasis incidence:**
    - In the control group, 95% of children developed atelectasis immediately after intubation compared to 52% in the CPAP group.
2. **Improved lung aeration:**
    - The CPAP group showed significantly lower lung ultrasound (LUS) aeration scores (3.5 vs. 8.8 in the control group), indicating better lung expansion.
3. **Enhanced oxygenation:**
    - CPAP minimized the shunt effect caused by alveolar collapse, maintaining SpO_2 levels during induction.

Effects of CPAP during emergence

1. **Lower postoperative atelectasis:**
    - Residual atelectasis was observed in only 10% of the CPAP group, compared to 30% in the control group.
2. **Sustained lung aeration:**
    - Aeration scores remained better in the CPAP group one hour after surgery (0.5 vs. 2.5), reflecting prolonged benefits.
3. **Minimized recruitment maneuvers:**
    - Children in the CPAP group required fewer recruitment maneuvers, reducing potential complications and procedural delays.

Implementing CPAP in pediatric anesthesia

Practical protocol

1. **Induction phase:**
    - Apply 5 cmH_2O of CPAP during mask ventilation with an FIO_2 of 1.0 for safety.
    - Mechanical ventilation with CPAP should be used immediately after intubation to maintain lung expansion.
2. **Emergence phase:**
    - Continue CPAP during the transition from mechanical ventilation to spontaneous breathing.
    - Maintain a moderate PEEP of 5-8 cmH_2O until extubation.
3. **Lung recruitment maneuvers:**
    - Use recruitment maneuvers selectively for children who develop atelectasis despite CPAP. Maintain pressures of up to 30 cmH_2O for 10 breaths to reopen collapsed alveoli.

Equipment and monitoring

1. **CPAP systems:**
    - Modern anesthesia workstations are equipped to deliver CPAP during both spontaneous and controlled ventilation.
    - Ensure compatibility with pediatric circuits and masks.
2. **Lung ultrasound (LUS):**
    - Use LUS for real-time assessment of lung aeration and detection of atelectasis.
    - Incorporate LUS into standard protocols for perioperative respiratory monitoring.

Benefits of CPAP

1. **Improved perioperative outcomes:**
   - CPAP reduces atelectasis, leading to better oxygenation and fewer pulmonary complications.
2. **Minimized interventions:**
   - Preventive CPAP decreases the need for recruitment maneuvers, reducing procedure-related risks.
3. **Enhanced recovery:**
   - Lower postoperative atelectasis contributes to faster recovery and improved patient comfort.

Limitations

- **Study population:**
  - The findings from Acosta et al. (2021) are limited to healthy children (ASA PS I). Further research is needed to evaluate CPAP's efficacy in high-risk populations, such as those with respiratory comorbidities.
- **Individualized approaches:**
  - The study used a fixed CPAP level of 5 cmH_2O. Future studies should explore tailored CPAP settings based on patient-specific factors, such as age, weight, and surgical type.

Key takeaways

☑ Atelectasis is a common and preventable complication during pediatric anesthesia.

☑ Continuous positive airway pressure (5 cmH_2O) during induction and emergence significantly reduces atelectasis and improves lung aeration.

☑ CPAP minimizes the need for intraoperative recruitment maneuvers and lowers the incidence of residual postoperative atelectasis.

☑ Implementation of CPAP requires appropriate equipment, structured protocols, and the integration of lung ultrasound for real-time monitoring.

Additional recommended reading:

1. Acosta CM, Lopez Vargas MP, Oropel F, et al. Prevention of atelectasis by continuous positive airway pressure in anaesthetized children: a randomized controlled study. *Eur J Anaesthesiol.* 2021;38(1):41-48. PMID: 33009190.
2. Von Ungern-Sternberg BS, Regli A, Schibler A, et al. The impact of positive end-expiratory pressure on functional residual capacity and ventilation homogeneity impairment in anesthetized children exposed to high levels of inspired oxygen. *Anesth Analg.* 2007;104:1364-1368. PMID: 17513627.
3. Song IK, Kim EH, Lee JH, et al. Effects of an alveolar recruitment maneuver guided by lung ultrasound on anesthesia-induced atelectasis in infants: a randomized controlled trial. *Anaesthesia.* 2016;72:214-222. PMID: 27804117.

Airway management in neonates and infants

07

Why this topic is important

Airway management in neonates and infants poses unique challenges due to their distinct anatomy, physiology, and vulnerability to complications. Neonates and infants are at high risk for adverse airway events, including hypoxemia, airway trauma, and respiratory failure, making proper preparation and management critical. Current guidelines for airway management in these populations have historically been limited, leaving clinicians without a standardized framework.

Recognizing this gap, the European Society of Anaesthesiology and Intensive Care (ESAIC) and the British Journal of Anaesthesia (BJA) collaborated to produce evidence-based guidelines to assist anesthesiologists in optimizing airway management in this vulnerable group. This update presents the key recommendations from these guidelines.

Objectives of this update

- Summarize evidence-based strategies for airway management in neonates and infants.
- Highlight best practices and key techniques for preoperative preparation, intubation, extubation, and managing difficult airways.
- Provide actionable recommendations for improving safety and outcomes in pediatric airway management.

What is new

This guideline[1] consolidates evidence from over a decade of research, addressing seven critical areas of airway management, including videolaryngoscopy, pharmacological preparation, difficult airway algorithms, and post-extubation care. It also introduces structured frameworks and recommendations based on the GRADE methodology, specifically for neonates and infants.

Key recommendations for neonatal and infant airway management

Preoperative airway assessment

- **Recommendation:** Use medical history and physical examination to predict difficult airway management (GRADE: 1C).
    - Although data on neonates and infants is limited, physical features such as craniofacial abnormalities, limited mouth opening, or cervical spine abnormalities should prompt enhanced preparation.
    - Syndromes such as Pierre Robin, Treacher-Collins, and Down syndrome are associated with airway challenges and should be identified during the preoperative assessment.

Pharmacological preparation

- **Sedation and anesthesia:** Adequate sedation or general anesthesia is critical to ensuring safety and comfort during airway management (GRADE: 1B).
- **Neuromuscular blocking agents (NMBAs):** Recommended for tracheal intubation unless spontaneous breathing is necessary (GRADE: 1C).
    - NMBAs improve intubation conditions and reduce complications such as laryngospasm. Rocuronium at low doses (e.g., 0.2 mg/kg) has shown efficacy in improving first-pass success rates.

Tracheal intubation techniques

- **Videolaryngoscopy (VL):**
    - Recommended as the first-choice technique for intubation in neonates and infants (GRADE: 1B). It improves glottic visualization and first-pass success rates compared to direct laryngoscopy.
    - VL is also effective for teaching and should be a standard tool in anesthesia suites, intensive care units, and emergency departments.
    - Apneic oxygenation during intubation is recommended to reduce the risk of desaturation, especially in neonates (GRADE: 1B).

Difficult airway management

- **Anticipated difficult airways:**
    - At least one VL, a flexible bronchoscope, and a supraglottic airway device (SGA) should be readily available.
    - Limit intubation attempts to reduce complications; consider changing technique or operator after each failed attempt (GRADE: 1C).
- **Unanticipated difficulties:**
    - A cognitive aid or algorithm for neonatal and infant airway management is essential to standardize responses and reduce adverse events.
- **Rescue oxygenation:**
    - SGAs are strongly recommended when intubation or mask ventilation fails (GRADE: 1B).

Confirmation of tracheal intubation

- **Gold standard:** Bilateral chest auscultation and end-tidal CO_2 waveform are recommended to confirm successful intubation (GRADE: 1C).
    - In complex cases, ultrasonography or videolaryngoscopy can supplement confirmation techniques.
    - Chest X-rays remain the gold standard for ensuring proper tube placement, though ultrasonography is gaining popularity for real-time confirmation.

Post-extubation strategies

- **Respiratory support:** High-flow nasal oxygenation (HFNO), continuous positive airway pressure (CPAP), or nasal intermittent positive pressure ventilation (NIPPV) should be used to prevent extubation failure (GRADE: 1B).

- **Extubation timing:**
    - Awake extubation is recommended for high-risk cases to avoid complications like laryngospasm or airway obstruction.
    - If deep extubation is chosen, it should only be performed by experienced providers with resources for immediate reintubation.

Human factors and training

- Human factors, such as teamwork and communication, play a crucial role in successful airway management.
- Simulation-based training is recommended to improve both technical and non-technical skills in pediatric airway management.

Implementation considerations

- **Training and education:** Implementing these guidelines requires widespread education and hands-on training in pediatric airway techniques, especially VL and flexible bronchoscopy.
- **Resources and equipment:** Ensure that appropriate airway devices, including age-specific VL blades, SGAs, and bronchoscopes, are readily available in all settings where neonates and infants are treated.
- **Institutional protocols:** Use these guidelines as a basis for creating or updating local standard operating procedures for pediatric airway management.

Key takeaways

☑ Neonates and infants require unique approaches to airway management due to their distinct anatomical and physiological characteristics.

☑ Videolaryngoscopy is the preferred first-line intubation technique, improving success rates and safety.

☑ Structured preparation, including pharmacological strategies and cognitive aids, reduces complications and enhances outcomes.

☑ Limiting intubation attempts and having a clear algorithm for managing difficulties is essential for patient safety.

☑ Post-extubation respiratory support and careful timing of extubation are critical to prevent failure.

☑ Human factors, including teamwork and structured training, are integral to improving airway management outcomes.

Additional recommended reading:

1. Disma N, Asai T, Cools E, et al. Airway management in neonates and infants: European Society of Anaesthesiology and Intensive Care and British Journal of Anaesthesia joint guidelines. *Br J Anaesth.* 2024;132(1):124-144. PMID: 38065762.
2. Cook TM, Woodall N, Frerk C. Major complications of airway management in the UK: results of the Fourth National Audit Project. *Br J Anaesth.* 2011;106(5):617-631. PMID: 21447488.
3. Matava CT, Kovatsis PG, Summers JL, et al. Pediatric airway management in COVID-19 patients: Consensus guidelines from the Society for Pediatric Anesthesia's Pediatric Difficult Intubation Collaborative and the Canadian Pediatric Anesthesia Society. *Anesth Analg.* 2020;131(1):61-73. PMID: 32287142; PMCID: PMC7173403.

Difficult neonatal airway management during pyloric stenosis repair

08

Why this topic is important

Managing the airway of neonates undergoing surgical repair for hypertrophic pyloric stenosis (HPS) presents significant challenges. These neonates often appear healthy but face unique risks during anesthesia, including pulmonary aspiration, hypoxemia, and difficult intubation. This combination of factors demands precise preparation and execution of airway management techniques.

HPS, characterized by gastric outlet obstruction, necessitates urgent surgical intervention. Anesthesia for HPS repair is further complicated by the need to manage a "full stomach" and rapidly desaturating patients with limited physiological reserves. These complexities make HPS an essential focus for airway safety improvements in neonatal care. Findings from the NECTARINE study[1] (NEonate and Children audiT of Anaesthesia pRactice IN Europe) highlight the elevated risk of difficult airway management in these patients, underscoring the need for tailored strategies to reduce complications and optimize outcomes.

Objectives of this update

- Summarize the specific challenges and risks of airway management in neonates undergoing HPS repair.
- Discuss evidence-based strategies for managing induction, intubation, and complications in this vulnerable population.
- Emphasize the importance of preparation, senior expertise, and institutional protocols in mitigating risks.

What is new

The NECTARINE study, a multicenter European audit, provides robust data comparing neonates undergoing HPS repair with those undergoing other surgeries. Key findings include:

- A 7.96% incidence of difficult airway management during HPS repair, nearly double the 4.41% incidence in non-HPS neonatal surgeries.
- Comparable rates of hypoxemia between HPS and other cases linked to induction techniques rather than the surgical condition itself.
- Insights into induction strategies, including modified rapid-sequence induction (RSI) and neuromuscular blockade, which can mitigate the risk of airway complications.

Airway challenges in pyloric stenosis repair

Patient-specific risks

Neonates with HPS are typically 1-2 months old and weigh around 3-4 kg. While generally free of significant comorbidities, their unique physiological and anatomical features contribute to increased perioperative risks:

- **Pulmonary aspiration:** Due to gastric outlet obstruction, these patients have a "full stomach," increasing the likelihood of regurgitation during induction.
- **Hypoxemia:** Neonates desaturate rapidly because of their high oxygen consumption and low functional residual capacity. Without proper preoxygenation and airway techniques, this can occur within seconds.
- **Difficult intubation:** The combination of anatomical considerations (e.g., a larger tongue and smaller airway) and suboptimal conditions during RSI can lead to challenges in securing the airway.

Induction techniques and airway management

- **Rapid-sequence induction (RSI):**
  - Classical RSI, which involves no mask ventilation before intubation, is often employed to minimize aspiration risk in HPS cases.
  - However, this technique increases the like-lihood of hypoxemia and multiple intubation attempts, particularly if preoxygenation is inadequate.
  - Modified RSI, incorporating gentle mask ventilation, allows for oxygenation without significantly increasing aspiration risk, improving outcomes in this population.
- **Neuromuscular blockade:**
  - Used in 92.3% of cases during the NECTARINE study, neuromuscular blocking agents (NMBAs) optimize intubation conditions by reducing muscle tone and improving visualization of the glottis.
  - The absence of NMBA was associated with higher rates of failed intubation and airway trauma, emphasizing its importance during RSI.
- **Videolaryngoscopy (VL):**
  - VL is increasingly recognized as the preferred tool for neonatal intubation. It offers superior glottic visualization and reduces the number of intubation attempts compared to direct laryngoscopy (DL).
  - For HPS cases, where first-pass success is crucial, VL provides a significant safety advantage.

Outcomes and complications

1. **Difficult airway management:**
   - Defined as more than two unsuccessful intubation attempts requiring a change in technique or additional assistance.
   - Occurred in 7.96% of HPS repair cases, significantly higher than the 4.41% seen in non-HPS surgeries.
2. **Hypoxemia during induction:**
   - Incidence was comparable between HPS cases (3.82%) and non-HPS cases (3.63%), indicating that induction techniques, rather than the surgical condition, play a central role.
   - Hypoxemia was often associated with class-ical RSI and inadequate preoxygenation.
3. **Postoperative outcomes:**
   - The NECTARINE cohort reported no mortality at 30 or 90 days following HPS repair.
   - Postoperative compwlications were rare (5.6%) and predominantly surgical, including the need for reoperations.

Strategies to improve safety in HPS repair

Preparation and preoperative planning

- **Risk assessment:**
  - Conduct thorough evaluations of airway and medical history, focusing on factors that may exacerbate airway challenges.
  - Collaboration with pediatric surgeons and neonatologists ensures optimal preoperative preparation, including correcting electrolyte imbalances and dehydration.
- **Institutional protocols:**
  - Establish standardized airway management pathways tailored to neonatal HPS cases, including modified RSI techniques and cognitive aids for managing complications.
  - Simulation training for anesthesia teams can improve response times and adherence to protocols in emergencies.

Induction and intubation best practices

- **Modified RSI:**
  - Incorporate gentle bag-mask ventilation during RSI to maintain oxygenation without significantly increasing aspiration risk.
  - Avoid classical RSI in cases where rapid desaturation is anticipated.
- **Optimal positioning:**
  - Neonates should be positioned with a shoulder roll to align the oral, pharyngeal, and laryngeal axes for improved intubation conditions.
- **Neuromuscular blockade:**
  - Routine use of agents such as rocuronium or succinylcholine ensures better intubation conditions and reduces the risk of failed attempts.
- **Videolaryngoscopy:**
  - Use VL as the first-line intubation tool, particularly in high-risk cases or when anatomical challenges are anticipated.

Post-intubation care

- Confirm endotracheal tube placement with end-tidal CO_2 monitoring and auscultation.
- Post-extubation, provide high-flow oxygen therapy or CPAP to minimize respiratory complications, particularly in neonates with underlying vulnerabilities.

Key takeaways

- ☑ Neonates undergoing HPS repair face a nearly doubled risk of difficult airway management compared to those undergoing other surgeries.
- ☑ Classical RSI techniques contribute to hypoxemia and multiple intubation attempts; modified RSI and neuromuscular blockade should be prioritized to improve safety.
- ☑ Videolaryngoscopy enhances first-pass success rates and reduces complications, making it the preferred intubation technique for HPS repair.
- ☑ Institutional preparation, senior anesthesiologist involvement, and adherence to evidence-based protocols are critical for optimizing outcomes.
- ☑ Ongoing education, simulation training, and structured risk assessment are essential to improving care in this vulnerable population.

<u>**Additional recommended reading:**</u>

1. Disma N, Engelhardt T, Hansen TG, et al. Neonates undergoing pyloric stenosis repair are at increased risk of difficult airway management: secondary analysis of the NECTARINE study. *Br J Anaesth.* 2022;129(5):734-739. PMID: 36085092.
2. Engelhardt T, Virag K, Veyckemans F, et al. Airway management in paediatric anaesthesia in Europe: insights from APRICOT (Anaesthesia Practice in Children Observational Trial). *Br J Anaesth.* 2018;121(1):66-75. PMID: 29935596.
3. Park RS, Rattana-Arpa S, Peyton JM, et al. Risk of Hypoxemia by Induction Technique Among Infants and Neonates Undergoing Pyloromyotomy. *Anesth Analg.* 2021;132(2):367-373. PMID: 31361669.

Teaching neonatal airway management

09

Why this topic is important

Neonatal airway management is among the most technically demanding and high-stakes procedures in anesthesiology. Neonates are anatomically and physiologically distinct, with a high oxygen consumption rate, low functional residual capacity, and a compliant chest wall, making them more prone to hypoxemia and bradycardia during airway management. These factors make it essential to succeed on the first intubation attempt, as multiple attempts significantly increase the risk of severe complications, including cardiac arrest and ischemic brain injury.

Despite the critical nature of neonatal intubation, there are substantial gaps in formal training and standardization of teaching methods. Improving first-attempt success rates requires both technical proficiency and a comprehensive understanding of neonatal anatomy, physiology, and equipment. This update highlights strategies to enhance neonatal airway safety and improve training through structured education and the incorporation of simulation-based learning.

Objectives of this update

- Emphasize the importance of first-attempt success in neonatal airway management.
- Review strategies to optimize oxygenation, anesthesia depth, and equipment selection.
- Explore training methodologies, including simulation and competency-based education, to improve skills in neonatal intubation.

What is new

Recent advancements in neonatal airway management emphasize a multifaceted approach:

- Incorporation of videolaryngoscopy (VL) as a teaching tool to improve trainee success and reduce complications.
- Use of passive oxygenation techniques to prolong safe apnea time during intubation attempts.
- Human factors, including team communication and situational awareness, are critical components of airway safety.
- Development of structured, simulation-based training programs to build and assess competence in neonatal intubation.

Principles of neonatal airway management

Unique challenges in neonatal anatomy and physiology

Neonates differ significantly from older children and adults in their airway anatomy and respiratory physiology:

1. **Anatomical considerations:**
    - Larger occiput, leading to cervical flexion, which can obstruct the airway.
    - Cephalad and anterior larynx (at C2-C3), requiring precise blade positioning during laryngoscopy.
    - Narrow and angled epiglottis that can be challenging to displace.
2. **Physiological vulnerabilities:**
    - Increased oxygen consumption (6-8 mL/kg/min) and low functional residual capacity lead to rapid desaturation during apnea.
    - Immature airway reflexes, including a heightened risk of laryngospasm and bradycardia.
3. **High-risk scenarios:**
    - Neonates with congenital abnormalities, such as micrognathia or craniofacial syndromes, are particularly challenging to intubate.

Maintaining oxygenation during intubation

Oxygenation is the cornerstone of neonatal airway management:

1. **Preoxygenation:** Optimize oxygen reserves before intubation using a high-flow nasal cannula (HFNO) or tight-fitting facemasks with 100% oxygen.

2. **Passive oxygenation:** Deliver oxygen during laryngoscopy to prolong safe apnea time. HFNO and systems like THRIVE (transnasal humidified rapid-insufflation ventilatory exchange) have shown promise in maintaining oxygenation during apneic periods.

3. **Avoid prolonged attempts:** Limit intubation attempts to reduce the risk of severe hypoxemia.

Optimizing first-attempt success

Anesthetic depth and muscle relaxation

- Adequate sedation and anesthetic depth prevent adverse airway responses, such as laryngospasm.

- Neuromuscular blocking agents (NMBDs) improve intubation conditions and reduce complications. Evidence from multiple studies suggests that NMBD use increases success rates compared to spontaneous ventilation techniques.

Equipment selection

1. **Videolaryngoscopy (VL):**
    - Provides superior visualization of the glottis, improving first-pass success rates, especially in difficult airways.
    - Facilitates real-time coaching during training, enhancing skill acquisition among trainees.
2. **Blade selection:**
    - Straight blades (e.g., Miller) are preferred for neonatal intubation due to their ability to lift the epiglottis effectively.
    - Hyperangulated blades may be beneficial in cases with anterior glottis positioning.

Training for neonatal airway management

The role of simulation

Simulation-based education is transforming the training of neonatal airway management:

1. **Technical skill acquisition:**
    - Realistic manikins allow repeated practice of intubation techniques in a controlled environment, reducing reliance on clinical exposure.
2. **Competency-based assessments:**
    - Tools like the Neonatal Intubation Scoring Instrument (NISI) provide objective metrics for evaluating performance.
3. **Team training:**
    - Simulation emphasizes the importance of communication, role delegation, and situational awareness during airway emergencies.

Videolaryngoscopy as a teaching tool

Videolaryngoscopy is invaluable for teaching neonatal airway management:

- The shared view between the trainee and supervisor facilitates real-time coaching and corrective feedback.
- Studies show that VL improves trainee success rates and reduces complications compared to direct laryngoscopy.

Ongoing education and skill retention

- Regular booster sessions and refreshers using simulation ensure the retention of neonatal intubation skills, particularly in centers with limited neonatal caseloads.
- Emerging technologies, such as virtual reality (VR) and artificial intelligence (AI), offer innovative approaches to supplement traditional training.

Human factors and non-technical skills

Non-technical skills play a critical role in neonatal airway safety:

1. **Team dynamics:**
    - Clear communication and role allocation improve efficiency and reduce errors during intubation.
2. **Cognitive aids:**
    - Checklists and standardized protocols enhance preparedness and mitigate risks.
3. **Situational awareness:**
    - Maintaining focus and anticipating complications are key to successful airway management.

Key takeaways

☑ Every neonatal intubation should be considered a critical event, requiring meticulous preparation and execution.

☑ Strategies to improve first-attempt success include adequate preoxygenation, appropriate anesthetic depth, and careful device selection.

☑ Videolaryngoscopy improves visualization and facilitates teaching, making it the preferred tool for neonatal airway management.

☑ Simulation-based training enhances technical skills, teamwork, and situational awareness, bridging gaps in clinical exposure.

☑ Structured education and regular practice are essential to maintaining competence in neonatal airway management.

Additional recommended reading:

1. Garcia-Marcinkiewicz AG, Matava CT. Safe in the first attempt: teaching neonatal airway management. *Curr Opin Anesthesiol.* 2022;35:329-336. PMID: 35671020.

2. Foglia EE, Ades A, Sawyer T, et al. Neonatal intubation practice and outcomes: an international registry study. *Pediatrics.* 2019;143:e20180902. PMID: 30538147; PMCID: PMC6317557.

3. Fiadjoe JE, Nishisaki A, Jagannathan N, et al. Airway management complications in children with difficult tracheal intubation from the Pediatric Difficult Intubation (PeDI) registry: a prospective cohort analysis. *Lancet Respir Med.* 2016;4:37-48. PMID: 26705976.

Difficult facemask ventilation in children

10

Why this topic is important

Facemask ventilation is a vital component of pediatric airway management, particularly when tracheal intubation is difficult or impossible. Challenges in facemask ventilation are compounded by anatomical and physiological features unique to children, including low functional residual capacity (FRC), higher oxygen consumption, and craniofacial anomalies. These issues increase the risk of severe hypoxemia, airway trauma, and cardiac arrest if ventilation is not achieved promptly.

The Pediatric Difficult Intubation (PeDI) registry provides critical insights into the prevalence, risk factors, and effective management strategies for difficult or impossible facemask ventilation in pediatric patients.

Objectives of this update

- Identify risk factors and syndromic features associated with difficult or impossible facemask ventilation.
- Highlight evidence-based management strategies, including supraglottic airways (SGAs) and neuromuscular blocking agents (NMBAs).
- Provide actionable recommendations to optimize safety and outcomes during pediatric airway management.

What is new

A retrospective analysis of 5,453 cases from the PeDI registry revealed:

- The incidence of difficult facemask ventilation was 9%, with impossible ventilation reported in 1%.
- Syndromes like Treacher-Collins syndrome, Pierre Robin sequence, and Goldenhar syndrome remain leading causes of difficult ventilation.
- Effective management strategies included:
    - SGAs improving ventilation in 71% of difficult cases.
    - NMBAs maintaining ventilation in 90% of cases with functional obstructions.
- Inhalational induction facilitated smoother transitions to positive pressure ventilation in high-risk cases.

Prevalence and risk factors

Incidence

- Difficult facemask ventilation: 9%
- Impossible facemask ventilation: 1%

Patients with difficult ventilation had a threefold higher complication rate, including:

- Hypoxemia (25% vs. 7%)
- Cardiac arrest (6% vs. 0.4%)
- Severe airway trauma (3% vs. 0.5%)

Patient-specific risk factors

1. **Age and weight:**
    - Infants and children with weight extremes (< 5th or > 95th percentile) face increased risk.
    - Odds of difficult ventilation are 2.35 times higher in infants.
2. **Syndromes and physical anomalies:**
    - Conditions such as Treacher-Collins syndrome, Pierre Robin sequence, and Goldenhar syndrome were associated with the highest prevalence of difficult ventilation. Specific anatomical features contributing to these challenges include:
        - Glossoptosis
        - Micrognathia
        - Limited mouth opening
    - Other conditions and syndromes to consider include:
        - Neuromuscular diseases: Reduced muscle tone and weakness can impair airway patency and ventilation.
        - Cleft lip and palate: Anatomical disruptions that may complicate mask ventilation and intubation.
        - Down syndrome: Characterized by macroglossia, hypotonia, and subglottic stenosis, which can increase airway difficulty.
        - Laryngomalacia and Tracheomalacia: Airway collapsibility that can exacerbate ventilation challenges, particularly in infants and children.
3. **Physiological factors:**
    - Low FRC and higher oxygen consumption in children lead to rapid desaturation.
    - High respiratory rates and smaller reserves exacerbate hypoxia.
4. **Location and induction method:**
    - Intubations outside the operating room, particularly in ICUs, are associated with higher difficulty rates.
    - Inhalational induction facilitates a controlled transition from spontaneous to positive-pressure ventilation, reducing difficulties.

Management strategies to improve mask ventilation

Positioning

- Optimize head and neck position using the **"sniffing" position.**
- Use shoulder rolls in infants to align the airway.

Equipment

Ensure availability of:

- Appropriate mask sizes for a proper seal
- Video-assisted laryngoscopy
- Oral and nasal airways
- Second-generation SGAs for airway protection

Supraglottic airways (SGAs)

- SGAs were used in 34% of difficult ventilation cases and 57% of impossible ventilation cases.
- Ventilation improved in:
    - 71% of cases with difficult facemask ventilation.
    - 48% of cases with impossible facemask ventilation.
- SGAs are particularly useful in situations of functional airway obstruction, such as laryngospasm or bronchospasm.

Pharmacological interventions

- Neuromuscular blocking agents (NMBAs) were administered in 31% of difficult ventilation cases.
- In these cases, NMBAs:
  - Improved or maintained ventilation in 90% of patients with difficult facemask ventilation.
  - Improved or maintained ventilation in 86% of patients with impossible facemask ventilation.
- While effective, NMBAs should be used cautiously in anatomically obstructed airways where worsening of ventilation is a possibility.

Preoxygenation

Optimize oxygen reserves before induction using techniques such as high-flow nasal oxygen or a tight-sealing facemask.

Induction method

Favor inhalational induction in high-risk cases to allow a controlled transition to positive-pressure ventilation.

Team readiness

- Conduct simulation-based training for difficult airway scenarios.
- Ensure skilled personnel are prepared, with access to rescue devices and videolaryngoscopy systems.

Institutional protocols

- Develop standardized algorithms incorporating SGAs, NMBAs, and videolaryngoscopy.
- Implement protocols for non-OR settings, where ventilation challenges are more frequent.

Practical recommendations for clinicians

Risk stratification

- Evaluate preoperative risk factors such as age, weight, craniofacial anomalies, and syndromic features.
- Anticipate challenges in children with Treacher Collins syndrome, Pierre Robin sequence, and similar conditions.

Procedural adjustments

1. **SGAs as rescue devices:**
   - Use SGAs early in cases of difficult or impossible facemask ventilation.
   - Consider second-generation SGAs for better seal and airway protection.
2. **NMBAs for functional obstruction:**
   - Administer NMBAs to address functional obstructions, such as laryngospasm or chest wall rigidity, unless contraindicated.
3. **Choice of induction:**
   - Favor inhalational induction in high-risk cases to allow a more controlled transition to positive-pressure ventilation.

Key takeaways

- ☑ Difficult or impossible facemask ventilation occurs in 9% of pediatric patients with difficult intubation and is associated with increased morbidity.
- ☑ Syndromes like Treacher Collins and physical anomalies such as glossoptosis and limited mouth opening significantly increase risk.
- ☑ Supraglottic airways and neuromuscular blocking agents are effective tools for managing difficult ventilation but require judicious use.
- ☑ Anticipation, preparation, and adherence to evidence-based protocols are essential to minimize complications and improve outcomes.

Additional recommended reading:

1. Garcia-Marcinkiewicz AG, Lee LK, Haydar B, et al. Difficult or impossible facemask ventilation in children with difficult tracheal intubation: a retrospective analysis of the PeDI registry. *Br J Anaesth.* 2023;131(1):178-187. PMID: 37076335.
2. Fiadjoe JE, Nishisaki A, Jagannathan N, et al. Airway management complications in children with difficult tracheal intubation from the PeDI registry: a prospective cohort analysis. *Lancet Respir Med.* 2016;4(1):37-48. PMID: 26705976.
3. Black AE, Flynn PER, Smith HL, et al. Development of a guideline for the management of the unanticipated difficult airway in pediatric practice. *Pediatr Anaesth.* 2015;25(4):346-362. PMID: 25684039.

NYSORA

Advances in pediatric airway management

11

Why this topic is important

Pediatric airway management is a cornerstone of anesthesia and critical care, but it presents unique challenges compared to adult populations. Children's distinct anatomical and physiological characteristics, including smaller airways, rapid oxygen consumption, and reduced functional residual capacity, predispose them to a higher risk of airway complications. Perioperative adverse respiratory events (PARE) such as laryngospasm, bronchospasm, and desaturation account for 60-75% of all critical perioperative incidents, making airway management the leading cause of morbidity and mortality in pediatric anesthesia.

Advances in technology, training, and evidence-based frameworks are transforming pediatric airway management. This update reviews these innovations, emphasizing their application in both routine and challenging scenarios. By integrating these practices, clinicians can improve safety and outcomes for this vulnerable population.

Objectives of this update

- Summarize the latest challenges and solutions in pediatric airway management.
- Highlight the benefits of videolaryngoscopy (VL), high-flow nasal oxygenation (HFNO), and apneic oxygenation in improving outcomes.
- Explore simulation-based training and artificial intelligence (AI) as tools for skill enhancement and decision support.
- Provide actionable recommendations to optimize care for pediatric patients.

What is new

Recent studies have provided critical insights into pediatric airway management:

- Videolaryngoscopy improves first-pass success rates, particularly in small infants and children with difficult airways.
- High-flow nasal oxygenation extends safe apnea time during intubation, reducing the risk of hypoxemia.
- Simulation training using advanced 3D models and machine learning is revolutionizing education and preparedness in pediatric airway management.

Addressing challenges in pediatric airway management

Unique anatomical and physiological considerations

Pediatric airway anatomy and physiology differ significantly from adults, making airway management more complex:

1. **Anatomy:**
   - The pediatric airway is smaller, funnel-shaped, and more anterior, with a relatively larger tongue and a narrow cricoid ring that serves as the narrowest part of the airway.
   - The larynx is higher in the neck (C3-C4), making visualization during laryngoscopy more challenging.
2. **Physiology:**
   - Children consume oxygen at 6-8 mL/kg/min, nearly twice the rate of adults, and have a smaller functional residual capacity.
   - These factors lead to rapid desaturation during apnea, necessitating efficient and timely airway interventions.

High-risk populations

Certain groups of children are at greater risk for airway complications:

- **Neonates and infants (< 1 year):** Their small airways and limited oxygen reserves make them particularly vulnerable.
- **Children with syndromes:** Conditions like Pierre Robin sequence, Treacher Collins syndrome, and mucopolysaccharidoses are associated with difficult airways due to craniofacial abnormalities.
- **Patients with respiratory conditions:** Children with asthma, bronchopulmonary dysplasia, or recent upper respiratory infections are more likely to experience perioperative respiratory complications.

Evidence-based tools and techniques

Videolaryngoscopy

- **Advantages:**
  - VL offers better visualization of the glottis, improving first-pass success rates and reducing esophageal intubations.
  - It particularly benefits neonates and children with anterior airways or difficult anatomy.
- **Evidence:**
  - The VISI (Video Laryngoscopy in Small Infants) trial reported a first-pass success rate of 93% with VL compared to 88% with direct laryngoscopy (DL).
  - Standard blade VL outperformed hyperangulated blades in children weighing less than 5 kg, demonstrating the importance of device selection.
- **Applications:**
  - VL is recommended as the first-line tool for both routine and difficult intubations in pediatric patients.

High-flow nasal oxygenation (HFNO)

- **Mechanism:**
  - HFNO delivers heated, humidified oxygen at high flow rates, maintaining oxygenation during apnea and prolonging the safe apnea time. An important variant of HFNO is Transnasal Humidified Rapid-Insufflation Ventilatory Exchange (THRIVE), which enhances the efficiency of oxygenation and ventilation during apneic episodes.
- **Benefits:**
  - HFNO, including THRIVE, doubles the duration of safe apnea compared to standard low-flow oxygen delivery, particularly in infants and children at risk of rapid desaturation.
- **Applications:**
  - HFNO, and specifically THRIVE, is ideal during prolonged intubation attempts, airway surgery, or in children with reduced oxygen reserves.

Apneic oxygenation

- **Low-flow oxygen:**
  - A simple, effective method to deliver oxygen during apnea, extending the safe window for intubation in children.
- **Indications:**
  - Recommended for high-risk airway cases, particularly when desaturation risk is high.
- **Limitations:**
  - Less effective in scenarios with significant intrapulmonary shunting, where oxygenation is compromised despite adequate ventilation.

Leveraging simulation and AI in pediatric airway management

Simulation-based training

Simulation offers a safe, controlled environment for skill acquisition and improvement:

- **Challenges in traditional models:**
  - Conventional pediatric airway mannequins often fail to replicate complex anatomical variations and dynamic airway conditions.
- **Advances:**
  - 3D-printed models simulate realistic pediatric airways, including those with congenital anomalies.
  - High-fidelity scenarios enhance both technical and non-technical skills, such as teamwork and crisis management.
- **Evidence:**
  - Simulation training has improved first-pass success rates and reduced complications in pediatric airway management.

Artificial intelligence and machine learning

- **Applications:**
  - AI algorithms are being developed to assist clinicians in identifying airway anatomy during laryngoscopy and bronchoscopy.
  - Real-time decision support tools are being explored to guide clinicians through complex airway scenarios.
- **Future potential:**
  - Integrating AI with VL could provide automated feedback, enhance accuracy, and reduce errors during intubation.

System-based approaches to improving pediatric airway management

Universal pediatric airway framework

To standardize care, a pediatric-specific framework separates oxygenation and ventilation management from intubation attempts:

1. **Plan A:**
   - Use advanced tools like VL and flexible bronchoscopes after two failed intubation attempts.
2. **Plan B:**
   - Switch to a supraglottic airway device (SGA) or use an alternative oxygenation strategy.
3. **Key focus:**
   - Maintain continuous oxygenation and ventilation throughout attempts to minimize complications.

Interdisciplinary collaboration

- **Airway teams:**
  - Hospitals should establish multidisciplinary difficult airway services to ensure preparedness and quality improvement.

- **Team training:**
  - Regular simulation sessions for entire airway teams improve communication, role clarity, and overall outcomes during emergencies.

Practical recommendations for clinicians

Preparation

- Conduct thorough airway assessments to identify high-risk patients and plan for contingencies.
- Ensure availability of advanced airway tools, such as VL, HFNO, and SGAs.

Technique

- Use videolaryngoscopy as the first-line intubation tool for routine and difficult pediatric airways.
- Employ HFNO or other form of apneic oxygenation during prolonged intubation attempts to reduce desaturation risk.

Education and training

- Incorporate simulation-based training into institutional programs to improve skill retention and preparedness.
- Explore AI tools and advanced technologies to augment real-time clinical decision-making.

Key takeaways

☑ Pediatric airway management requires tailored strategies that address unique anatomical and physiological challenges.

☑ Videolaryngoscopy improves first-pass success rates and should be the standard of care in both routine and difficult cases.

☑ High-flow nasal oxygenation and apneic oxygenation are essential tools for maintaining oxygenation during intubation.

☑ Simulation and AI are transforming education and decision-making, enhancing both practitioner readiness and patient safety.

☑ A standardized framework and interdisciplinary collaboration are critical for achieving the best outcomes in pediatric airway management.

Additional recommended reading:

1. Hsu G, von Ungern-Sternberg BS, Engelhardt T. Advances in pediatric airway management: a systematic review. *Curr Opin Anesthesiol.* 2021;34(3):276-283. PMID: 33935175
2. Garcia-Marcinkiewicz AG, Kovatsis PG, Hunyady AI, et al. First-attempt success rate of video laryngoscopy in small infants (VISI): a multicenter randomized controlled trial. *Lancet.* 2020;396:1905-1913. PMID: 33308472.
3. Patel A, Nouraei SA. Transnasal humidified rapid-insufflation ventilatory exchange (THRIVE): a physiological method of increasing apnea time in patients with difficult airways. *Anaesthesia.* 2015;70(3):323-329. PMID: 25388828; PMCID: PMC4674986.
4. Disma N, Asai T, Cools E, et al. Airway management in neonates and infants: European Society of Anaesthesiology and Intensive Care and British Journal of Anaesthesia joint guidelines. *Eur J Anaesthesiol.* 2024;41(1):3-23 PMID: 38018248; PMCID: PMC10720842.
5. Krishna SG, Bryant JF, Tobias JD. Management of the Difficult Airway in the Pediatric Patient. *J Pediatr Intensive Care.* 2018;7(3):115-125. PMID: 31073483; PMCID: PMC6260357.

Predicting obstructive sleep apnea and perioperative respiratory risks in children

12

Why this topic is important

Obstructive sleep apnea (OSA) is a significant perioperative risk factor in pediatric patients, particularly those undergoing procedures like adenotonsillectomy. This condition, marked by the collapse of the upper airway during sleep, is associated with a higher likelihood of respiratory complications during and after anesthesia. Despite its prevalence, routine preoperative screening for OSA using polysomnography (PSG) is not widely performed due to resource limitations, leaving many cases undiagnosed.

The measurement of upper airway collapsibility, specifically through pharyngeal closing pressure (PCLOSE), has emerged as a promising alternative for identifying OSA severity in anesthetized children. This approach could transform perioperative risk assessments by providing a quick, non-invasive, and resource-efficient method for evaluating airway vulnerability and stratifying patient risk.

Objectives of this update

- Highlight the importance of assessing upper airway collapsibility for identifying OSA in pediatric patients.
- Examine the predictive utility of PCLOSE for both OSA and perioperative respiratory adverse events (PRAEs).
- Provide insights into the practical application of PCLOSE measurements in pediatric perioperative care.

What is new

- PCLOSE demonstrated high sensitivity (100%) for identifying moderate-to-severe OSA at a threshold of -4 cm H_2O.
- Children with moderate-to-severe OSA had significantly higher PCLOSE values, reflecting more easily collapsible airways.
- There was no significant correlation between PCLOSE and the occurrence of PRAEs, suggesting that collapsibility measurements alone may not predict respiratory complications.

Key findings

Study design

The prospective study by Ohn et al. 2023 involved 52 children undergoing elective adenotonsillectomy. Each participant underwent PSG prior to surgery to confirm OSA severity and had their PCLOSE measured while under general anesthesia. PRAEs were monitored and documented during the perioperative period.

Upper airway collapsibility and OSA prediction

- PCLOSE values were significantly less ne-gative in children with moderate-to-severe OSA compared to those with mild or no OSA.
- At a PCLOSE threshold of -4 cm H_2O, sensitivity for identifying moderate-to-severe OSA was 100%, with a specificity of 64.7%.
- The study revealed an excellent diagnostic ability for PCLOSE, with an area under the curve (AUC) of 0.857.

Upper airway collapsibility and PRAEs

- 56% of children experienced PRAEs, with airway obstruction, desaturation, and stridor being the most common.
- While collapsibility was more frequent in children who experienced PRAEs (60% vs. 40%), no statistically significant association was found between PCLOSE values and respiratory complications.
- The findings underscore that factors beyond airway collapsibility, such as comorbid conditions and perioperative management strategies, likely contribute to PRAEs.

Recommendations for practice

Integrating PCLOSE into perioperative care

1. Preoperative risk stratification:
   - Use PCLOSE as an adjunct to clinical evaluations to identify moderate-to-severe OSA in children, particularly in resource-limited settings where PSG is unavailable.
   - A PCLOSE value of > -4 cm H_2O can be a reliable threshold for identifying high-risk patients requiring enhanced perioperative monitoring.
2. Tailoring perioperative management:
   - Adjust anesthesia protocols for children identified with moderate-to-severe OSA to minimize respiratory complications.
   - Consider extubating these patients in a monitored setting and ensuring immediate availability of resuscitation equipment.
3. Education and training:
   - Train anesthesiology teams on PCLOSE measurements and their interpretation to enhance this method's clinical utility.
   - Emphasize the importance of multi-disciplinary collaboration between anesthe-siologists, surgeons, and sleep specialists in managing high-risk pediatric patients.

Addressing limitations of PCLOSE

- While PCLOSE reliably identifies OSA severity, it cannot independently predict PRAEs. Supplement collapsibility assessments with comprehensive evaluations of patient history, comorbidities, and surgical factors.
- Further research is needed to refine PCLOSE cutoffs for differentiating between OSA severities and to explore its role in broader pediatric populations with complex health profiles.

Broader implications

The study highlights PCLOSE's potential as a practical, efficient tool for perioperative OSA risk stratification in children. By identifying high-risk patients early, clinicians can implement targeted interventions to mitigate complications. However, its lack of predictive value for PRAEs suggests the need for a multimodal approach to perioperative risk assessment.

Future directions include:

- Developing automated systems for real-time PCLOSE analysis to enhance accessibility and accuracy.
- Conducting large-scale, multicenter studies to validate findings across diverse patient populations.
- Integrating collapsibility measurements into standard perioperative monitoring protocols for personalized anesthesia care.

Key takeaways

☑ Pharyngeal closing pressure (PCLOSE) offers a reliable, rapid method for identifying moderate-to-severe OSA in anesthetized children.

☑ At a threshold of -4 cm H_2O, PCLOSE achieves 100% sensitivity for moderate-to-severe OSA but cannot reliably predict perioperative respiratory adverse events.

☑ While useful for OSA risk stratification, PCLOSE should be complemented by thorough clinical assessments to guide perioperative management.

☑ Implementing PCLOSE measurements in routine practice could enhance perioperative safety and facilitate personalized care for pediatric patients.

Additional recommended reading:

1. Ohn M, Sommerfield D, Nguyen J, et al. Predicting obstructive sleep apnea and perioperative respiratory adverse events in children: role of upper airway collapsibility measurements. *Br J Anaesth.* 2023;131(6):1043-1052. PMID: 37891122.
2. Hillman DR, Walsh JH, Maddison KJ, et al. Evolution of changes in upper airway collapsibility during slow induction of anesthesia with propofol. *Anesthesiology.* 2009;111:63-71. PMID: 19512872.
3. von Ungern-Sternberg BS, Davies K, Hegarty M, et al. The effect of deep vs. awake extubation on respiratory complications in high-risk children undergoing adenotonsillectomy. *Eur J Anaesthesiol.* 2013;30:529-536. PMID: 23344124.

Apneic oxygenation during pediatric intubation

13

Why this topic is important

Tracheal intubation is a high-stakes procedure in pediatric anesthesia and critical care, often performed in situations where time and precision are critical. Unlike adults, neonates and young children have unique physiological vulnerabilities that increase their risk during intubation. Specifically, they have a smaller functional residual capacity, higher oxygen consumption, and lower oxygen reserves, leading to rapid desaturation during apnea. These factors contribute to a narrow window of safety, placing them at a higher risk of complications, including hypoxemia, bradycardia, and cardiac arrest.

Apneic oxygenation has emerged as an innovative strategy to improve safety during intubation. By delivering oxygen continuously during apnea, apneic oxygenation prolongs the safe apnea time, allowing more time for clinicians to perform intubation while maintaining oxygenation levels. Despite its promise, the adoption of this technique remains inconsistent, and its role in pediatric practice is under debate. A recent systematic review by Fuchs et al. consolidates existing evidence, highlighting its benefits and providing a roadmap for implementation in pediatric airway management.

Objectives of this update

- Summarize the evidence for apneic oxygenation in pediatric tracheal intubation.
- Discuss its impact on first-pass success, oxygen saturation, and adverse events during intubation.
- Provide practical guidance for the clinical application of apneic oxygenation in pediatric airway management.

What is new

The systematic review and meta-analysis conducted by Fuchs et al. included data from 15 studies with a total of 9,802 pediatric patients. This review comprehensively analyzes apneic oxygenation's effectiveness during tracheal intubation. Key findings include:

- **Improved first-pass success rates:** Apneic oxygenation increased first-pass success by 27%.
- **Reduced hypoxemia incidence:** The incidence of hypoxemia decreased by 76%.
- **Higher oxygen saturation levels:** Patients who received apneic oxygenation had an average oxygen saturation increase of 3.6% compared to those who did not.

These findings provide compelling evidence for the integration of apneic oxygenation into pediatric airway management protocols.

Benefits of apneic oxygenation in pediatric intubation

Prolonged safe apnea time

Safe apnea time refers to the duration between the cessation of ventilation and the critical drop in arterial oxygen saturation (SpO_2). In pediatric patients, this time is significantly shorter due to their high metabolic rate and limited oxygen reserves. Apneic oxygenation extends this window by maintaining oxygen delivery during apnea, giving clinicians additional time to secure the airway.

Improved first-pass intubation success

The meta-analysis demonstrated a 27% higher likelihood of first-pass intubation success with apneic oxygenation. First-pass success is critical because multiple intubation attempts increase the risk of complications, including airway trauma, aspiration, and hypoxemia. Enhanced success rates with apneic oxygenation contribute to safer and more efficient airway management.

Reduced risk of hypoxemia

Hypoxemia, defined as $SpO_2 < 90\%$, is a frequent complication during pediatric intubation. The meta-analysis found that apneic oxygenation reduced the absolute risk of hypoxemia by 31%. By maintaining oxygenation throughout the apneic period, apneic oxygenation minimizes the risk of severe desaturation, even in high-risk cases.

Higher oxygen saturation

Pediatric patients who received apneic oxygenation maintained oxygen saturation levels that were, on average, 3.6% higher than those who did not. This small but clinically meaningful improvement can be critical in preventing hypoxic injury, especially in neonates and infants with limited oxygen reserves.

Methods of delivering apneic oxygenation

Low-flow oxygen delivery

Low-flow oxygen systems, such as standard nasal cannulas, are widely used for apneic oxygenation. They are simple, inexpensive, and effective for most pediatric patients. These systems deliver oxygen at flow rates typically between 2 and 6 liters per minute, depending on the patient's size and clinical condition.

High-flow nasal oxygen (HFNO)

High-flow nasal oxygen systems, such as Optiflow, deliver warmed, humidified oxygen at flow rates up to 60 liters per minute. HFNO is particularly effective in pediatric patients as it provides superior oxygen delivery and mild positive airway pressure, which helps maintain airway patency. While more resource-intensive, HFNO has been shown to offer better outcomes in high-risk patients compared to low-flow systems.

Integrated systems

Advanced airway management tools now integrate apneic oxygenation capabilities, such as:

- **Nasal cannula combined with laryngoscopy:** Simple and effective for maintaining oxygenation during laryngoscopy.
- **Oxygenating laryngoscopes:** Devices such as the Oxiport laryngoscope deliver oxygen directly through channels in the blade or handle, ensuring a continuous oxygen supply during intubation or airway visualization. This innovative design enhances both visualization of the airway and patient oxygenation, making it particularly useful in difficult airway scenarios or during prolonged intubation attempts.

Clinical recommendations for using apneic oxygenation

Pre-intubation preparation

1. **Preoxygenation:** Optimize oxygenation levels before intubation by delivering 100% oxygen using a tight-fitting facemask. Aim for an end-tidal oxygen concentration (Eto_2) of ≥ 90%.

2. **Device selection:** Choose the appropriate oxygen delivery system based on the patient's size, condition, and available resources. HFNO is preferred for neonates and infants with significant hypoxemia.

During intubation

1. **Continuous oxygen delivery:** Apply apneic oxygenation throughout the intubation process using a nasal cannula or HFNO. This is particularly important for high-risk patients.

2. **Team coordination:** Ensure all team members know the apneic oxygenation strategy and that equipment is readily available.

In emergency situations

1. **Rapid sequence induction (RSI):** Incorporate apneic oxygenation into RSI protocols to prevent rapid desaturation.

2. **Difficult airway cases:** Use advanced systems like oxygenating laryngoscopes or HFNO in cases with anticipated airway challenges.

Implementation challenges

- **Knowledge gaps:** Many clinicians must become more familiar with the technique and its benefits.
- **Resource constraints:** High-flow systems are not universally available, particularly in resource-limited settings.
- **Inconsistent evidence:** Variability in study designs and patient populations complicates the development of standardized protocols.

Key takeaways

☑ Apneic oxygenation effectively improves safety during pediatric tracheal intubation, particularly in neonates and critically ill children.

☑ It reduces hypoxemia, increases first-pass success rates, and prolongs safe apnea time.

☑ Both low-flow and high-flow systems are effective, but HFNO offers additional benefits, especially for high-risk patients.

☑ To optimize outcomes, clinicians should incorporate apneic oxygenation into routine and emergency intubation protocols, ensuring proper training and resource availability.

Additional recommended reading:

1. Fuchs A, Koepp G, Huber M, et al. Apnoeic oxygenation during paediatric tracheal intubation: a systematic review and meta-analysis. *Br J Anaesth.* 2024;132(2):392-406. PMID: 38030551.
2. Humphreys S, Lee-Archer P, Reyne G, et al. Transnasal humidified rapid-insufflation ventilatory exchange (THRIVE) prolongs safe apnoea time in children. *Anaesthesia.* 2017;72(4):534-539. PMID: 28100527.
3. Patel A, Nouraei SA. Transnasal humidified rapid-insufflation ventilatory exchange (THRIVE): a physiological method of increasing apnoea time in patients with difficult airways. *Anaesthesia.* 2015;70(3):323-329. PMID: 25388828; PMCID: PMC4674986
4. Mitterlechner T, Herff H, Hammel CW, et al. A dual-use laryngoscope to facilitate apneic oxygenation. *J Emerg Med.* 2015;48(1):103-107. PMID: 25308899.

Airway challenges in COVID-19 patients

Difficult airway management in COVID-19 patients

14

Why this topic is important

Airway management in patients with COVID-19 presents unique challenges due to the risk of viral transmission, potential respiratory distress, and the impact of the disease on airway anatomy and function. Managing airways in COVID-19 patients requires a balance between protecting healthcare workers (HCWs) and ensuring patient safety. Unlike standard scenarios, COVID-19 necessitates additional measures like optimized preoxygenation, strict personal protective equipment (PPE) use, and specialized intubation techniques to reduce aerosol generation and ensure safe, successful intubation.

Objectives of this update

- Review specific considerations for managing difficult airways in adult COVID-19 patients.
- Highlight protocols to minimize HCW exposure while maintaining high first-pass intubation success rates.
- Provide actionable guidance for preoxygenation, intubation strategies, post-intubation care, and continuous monitoring.

What is new

The COVID-19 pandemic has amplified the need for robust, multidisciplinary airway management protocols:

- Risk assessment of respiratory status, airway anatomy (e.g., Mallampati score), and comorbidities is emphasized.
- Videolaryngoscopy (VL) is prioritized for its ability to enhance visualization and reduce operator-patient proximity.
- Sedative-assisted preoxygenation with high-flow nasal cannula (HFNC) improves oxygen reserves while minimizing aerosolization.
- Scalpel-bougie-tube cricothyrotomy remains the preferred invasive technique for "cannot intubate, cannot oxygenate" (CICO) emergencies.

Practical recommendations

Risk assessment

- Evaluate the patient's respiratory status, prior intubation experiences, and comorbidities.
- Conduct airway assessments, including Mallampati scoring, to identify anticipated difficulties.

Multidisciplinary team

- Clearly define roles for team members, including:
    - Primary intubator
    - Bag-mask ventilation operator
    - Emergency response lead
- Assign a PPE "spotter" to oversee safety measures.

Safety measures

- Use personal protective equipment (PPE):
    - N95 masks, face shields, gowns, and gloves.
    - Powered air-purifying respirators (PAPR) if available.
- Follow strict donning/doffing protocols to reduce contamination risk.

Equipment preparation

- Standard airway equipment:
    - Functioning suction, laryngoscopes, endotracheal tubes (ETT) of different sizes, and oral/nasal airways.
- Ensure capnography and wide-bore cannulas for enhanced circulation.
- Use vaporized agents to minimize aerosolization.

Preoxygenation strategies

- Preoxygenate with a well-sealed face mask and HEPA filter, delivering 100% oxygen.
- Use HFNC to improve oxygenation while reducing aerosolization risk.
- Aim for $SpO_2 > 94\%$ or preoxygenate for 3 minutes if end-tidal oxygen monitoring is unavailable.

Intubation strategy

- Rapid Sequence Induction (RSI): Preferred for minimizing the apneic period and reducing aspiration risk.
    - Use neuromuscular blockers like succinylcholine or rocuronium to facilitate rapid intubation.
- Videolaryngoscopy (VL):
    - First-line technique for intubation to increase visualization and reduce exposure risk.
    - Use hyper-angulated blades cautiously to avoid ETT passage challenges.
- Keep spontaneous ventilation if difficulty is anticipated before RSI.
- Bougie and awake fiberoptic intubation are options for failed visualizations.

Post-intubation management

- Use closed-circuit ventilation systems to minimize aerosolization.
- Avoid frequent suctioning; minimize circuit disconnections.
- Continuous monitoring:
    - Capnography (CO_2), SpO_2, and hemodynamic status.

Extubation considerations

- Perform awake extubation to ensure immediate reintubation capability if necessary.
- Reduce aerosol generation by:
    - Pre-medication with IV lidocaine or dexmedetomidine to suppress coughing.
    - Deep suctioning and HEPA filters to control aerosol spread.

Invasive airway management

- For "cannot intubate, cannot oxygenate" (CICO) emergencies:
  - Perform scalpel-bougie-tube cricothyrotomy as the preferred method.
- Avoid transtracheal jet ventilation due to aerosolization risks.

Key takeaways

☑ Airway management in COVID-19 patients requires a multidisciplinary approach with strict safety protocols to protect HCWs and optimize patient outcomes.

☑ Videolaryngoscopy is the preferred intubation technique, while HFNC preoxygenation minimizes hypoxia.

☑ Proper equipment preparation, PPE use, and post-intubation care are critical to reducing viral exposure and optimizing respiratory support.

☑ DSI may offer advantages in select patients requiring stabilization before intubation, improving preoxygenation and reducing complications.

Additional recommended reading:

1. Foley LJ, Urdaneta F, Berkow L, et al. Difficult airway management in adult coronavirus disease 2019 patients: statement by the Society of Airway Management. *Anesth Analg.* 2021;133(4):876-887. PMID: 33711004.
2. Cook TM, El-Boghdadly K, McGuire B, et al. Consensus guidelines for managing the airway in patients with COVID-19: recommendations from the difficult airway society and others. *Anaesthesia.* 2020;75(6):785-799. PMID: 32221970; PMCID: PMC7383579.
3. Wax RS, Christian MD. Practical recommendations for critical care teams caring for COVID-19 patients. *Can J Anaesth.* 2020;67(5):568-576. PMID: 32052373; PMCID: PMC7091420.

Airway challenges in critically ill COVID-19 patients

15

Why this topic is important

Airway management in critically ill COVID-19 patients presents a unique and formidable challenge for healthcare providers. These patients often experience severe hypoxemia, hemodynamic instability, and respiratory distress, conditions that significantly increase the risk of adverse events during intubation. Compounding these risks is the high transmissibility of SARS-CoV-2, which exposes clinicians to potential infection during aerosol-generating procedures like tracheal intubation.

The COVID-19 pandemic has highlighted the need for robust and tailored strategies to address these challenges. By leveraging lessons learned during the pandemic, clinicians can refine their airway management approaches for current and future respiratory crises. This update reviews the latest insights into preoxygenation, intubation techniques, hemodynamic optimization, and infection prevention in COVID-19.

Objectives of this update

- To summarize evidence-based strategies for airway management in critically ill COVID-19 patients.
- This study aims to assess the role of advanced techniques such as video laryngoscopy, noninvasive ventilation (NIV), and high-flow nasal oxygen (HFNO).
- To provide practical recommendations for minimizing complications and healthcare worker exposure.

Key challenges in airway management

1. Severe hypoxemia:
    - COVID-19 patients often present with profound oxygenation deficits, exacerbating the risk of hypoxemia during apnea and intubation.
    - Preoxygenation with NIV or HFNO is critical to mitigate these risks.
2. Hemodynamic instability:
    - Postintubation hypotension and cardiovascular collapse are common, driven by hypovolemia, high sympathetic drive, and induction agents.
3. High aerosolization risk:
    - Aerosol-generating procedures pose significant infection risks for healthcare workers, necessitating stringent personal protective equipment (PPE) protocols.
4. Complex intubations:
    - High rates of difficult intubation are associated with delayed first-pass success, increasing complications like aspiration and barotrauma.

Strategies for optimizing airway management

Preoxygenation and apneic oxygenation

Effective preoxygenation is essential for reducing peri-intubation hypoxemia.

1. NIV with HFNO:
   - Combining NIV with HFNO (OPTINIV) provides higher oxygen saturation and prolonged apnea times in severely hypoxemic patients.
   - This approach is especially beneficial in managing refractory hypoxemia.
2. Bag-mask ventilation:
   - Although associated with aerosolization, bag-mask ventilation may be cautiously applied using tight-fitting masks to prevent rapid desaturation.
3. Patient positioning:
   - Preoxygenation in an upright position improves functional residual capacity and oxygenation efficiency.

Intubation techniques

1. Videolaryngoscopy (VL):
   - VL reduces difficult intubations by improving glottic visualization and increasing the distance between the patient and the provider.
   - International guidelines recommend VL as the first-line tool for COVID-19 patients.
2. Rapid sequence induction (RSI):
   - RSI minimizes the duration of apnea and reduces the risk of aspiration.
   - Recommended agents include etomidate or ketamine combined with succinylcholine or rocuronium for neuromuscular blockade.
3. First-pass success:
   - Achieving first-pass intubation is critical to minimizing complications. Experienced providers should perform intubation whenever possible.

Hemodynamic optimization

Managing hemodynamic stability is crucial to prevent peri- and postintubation complications.

1. Preemptive measures:
   - Fluid resuscitation and vasopressors should be titrated based on volume responsiveness and systolic blood pressure thresholds (> 130 mmHg).
   - Continuous vasopressor infusions may be necessary during and after intubation.
2. Ventilation adjustments:
   - Use lung-protective strategies with low tidal volumes and positive end-expiratory pressure (PEEP) to prevent barotrauma and optimize oxygenation.

Infection prevention

Protecting healthcare workers during aerosol-generating procedures is a top priority.

1. PPE:
   - Adhere to institutional PPE protocols, including the use of powered air-purifying respirators (PAPRs) or N95 masks.
   - Double gloves, face shields, and full-body gowns are recommended for all intubation procedures.
2. Negative pressure rooms:
   - Conduct intubations in negative pressure rooms with a minimum of 12 air exchanges per hour to reduce airborne viral load.
3. Minimizing aerosolization:
   - Avoid unnecessary ventilator disconnections and use heat and moisture exchange filters to reduce viral spread.

Controversies and evolving insights

Timing of intubation

1. Early versus delayed intubation:
   - Conflicting evidence exists on the optimal timing for intubation. While early intubation may prevent clinical deterioration, delayed approaches using NIV and HFNO have shown similar survival outcomes in some studies.
2. ROX index:
   - The respiratory rate oxygenation index (ROX) helps predict the need for intubation. A threshold of > 5.37 is associated with reduced intubation risk.

Videolaryngoscopy outcomes

1. Operator expertise:
   - VL is most effective when performed by experienced operators. Training and simulation-based education are critical to improving first-pass success.
2. Stylet use:
   - The choice of adjuncts like stylets or bougies influences intubation success and should be tailored to individual patient anatomy.

Clinical recommendations

1. Preoxygenation:
   - Use NIV combined with HFNO for severely hypoxemic patients. Optimize patient positioning and monitor SpO_2 continuously.
2. Device selection:
   - Prioritize videolaryngoscopy for intubation and ensure operators are trained in its use.
3. Team preparation:
   - Designate roles, use checklists and ensure all necessary equipment is readily available before intubation.
4. Hemodynamic support:
   - Administer fluids and vasopressors proactively to maintain stable blood pressure and cardiac output.
5. Infection control:
   - Adhere to strict PPE protocols and conduct procedures in negative pressure environments to minimize healthcare worker exposure.

Key takeaways

- ☑ Airway management in COVID-19 patients is highly complex, with risks of hypoxemia, hemodynamic instability, and aerosolization.
- ☑ Advanced preoxygenation strategies like OPTINIV improve outcomes in severely hypoxemic patients.
- ☑ Videolaryngoscopy is recommended for intubation but requires experienced operators for optimal results.
- ☑ Hemodynamic optimization and infection prevention measures are essential to ensuring patient and provider safety.

Additional recommended reading:

1. De Jong A, Khanna AK. Airway management in the critically ill patient with COVID-19. *Curr Opin Anaesthesiol.* 2022;35:137-143. PMID: 35102046.

2. Cook TM, El-Boghdadly K, McGuire B, et al. Consensus guidelines for managing the airway in patients with COVID-19. *Anaesthesia*. 2020;75:785-799. PMID: 32221970; PMCID: PMC7383579.

3. Casey JD, Janz DR, Russell DW, et al. Bag-mask ventilation during tracheal intubation of critically ill adults. *N Engl J Med.* 2019;380:811-821. PMID: 30779528; PMCID: PMC6423976.

Controversies in airway management of COVID-19 patients

16

Why this topic is important

Airway management is a cornerstone of treating critically ill patients, particularly those with respiratory failure caused by COVID-19. Tracheal intubation and other aerosol-generating procedures (AGPs) pose significant risks for healthcare workers and demand precise protocols to ensure safety. The pandemic's evolving nature has prompted guidelines updates, reflecting lessons learned from global experiences.

The 2021 consensus recommendations by Wei et al. highlight strategies to optimize outcomes while mitigating risks. This update focuses on controversies in airway management, including personal protective equipment (PPE), high-flow nasal oxygen (HFNO), and the timing of tracheal intubation. These insights provide valuable guidance for healthcare providers navigating this complex landscape.

Objectives of this update

- Summarize expert consensus on key issues in airway management for COVID-19 patients.
- Discuss evidence-based recommendations for PPE use during AGPs.
- Examine the role of HFNO in respiratory support.
- Address controversies surrounding the timing of tracheal intubation.

What is new

- Clearer recommendations on using Level III PPE for high-risk AGPs like tracheal intubation.
- Evidence supports the cautious use of HFNO despite initial concerns about aerosol generation.
- Evolving perspectives on early versus delayed intubation, emphasizing individualized care.

Key findings

Personal protective equipment (PPE)

- Level III PPE: Provides the most effective protection for healthcare workers during AGPs, incorporating a powered air-purifying respirator (PAPR), a hooded coverall, and eye protection. Studies suggest zero infection rates among healthcare workers using this level of protection during intubation in COVID-19 patients.
- Global variability: Different regions employ varying PPE standards, leading to inconsistencies in infection rates. Level II PPE (e.g., N95 masks without full skin and eye protection) has been linked to higher infection rates.
- Fit testing and training: Proper PPE fit testing and supervised donning and doffing are crucial to minimize self-contamination risks.

Use of high-flow nasal oxygen (HFNO)

- Initial concerns: HFNO was initially avoided due to fears of aerosol generation and viral spread. Subsequent studies demonstrated no significant increase in transmission risk with proper use.
- Clinical benefits: HFNO can improve oxygenation and reduce the need for mechanical ventilation in selected patients, particularly those with mild to moderate respiratory failure.
- Implementation considerations: The use of HFNO requires additional precautions, including negative-pressure rooms and appropriate PPE, to ensure healthcare workers' safety.

Timing of tracheal intubation

- Early intubation: Advocated to prevent sudden deterioration and cross-infection risks associated with emergency intubations. Early intubation may also stabilize oxygenation and reduce hemodynamic compromise during induction.
- Delaying intubation: Emerging evidence suggests that delaying intubation in favor of HFNO or non-invasive ventilation (NIV) can benefit selected patients, particularly those with high lung compliance.
- Individualized approach: The decision to intubate should consider patient-specific factors, including respiratory mechanics, response to non-invasive support, and disease trajectory.

Challenges in airway management

Balancing safety and effectiveness

The primary challenge lies in balancing the need to protect healthcare workers and provide optimal patient care. This requires stringent infection control measures without compromising the speed and efficiency of airway interventions.

Resource disparities

Access to Level III PPE and advanced respiratory support devices remains unequal globally. Resource-constrained settings may face higher infection rates and limited options for non-invasive ventilation.

Inconsistent guidelines

Conflicting recommendations across different countries and institutions have created uncertainty regarding best practices, particularly in using HFNO and determining the timing of intubation.

Recommendations for improving outcomes

Strengthening infection control

- Universal adoption of Level III PPE: Ensure availability of comprehensive PPE for high-risk AGPs, with priority given to frontline workers in resource-limited settings.
- Standardized training: Implement universal protocols for PPE use, including regular fit testing and supervised donning/doffing.
- Dedicated isolation units: Ensure that all COVID-19 patients are treated in special isolation units to minimize transmission risks to healthcare workers and other patients.

Optimizing respiratory support

- Expanded HFNO use: Incorporate HFNO into treatment protocols for suitable patients, supported by clear guidance on safety measures and monitoring.
- Research investments: Support studies to clarify HFNO's role in managing COVID-19 and its long-term safety implications.

Guideline harmonization

- Foster international collaboration to align recommendations, reduce inconsistencies, and provide practical guidance for diverse healthcare settings.

Broader implications for future pandemics

The findings from this expert consensus have implications beyond COVID-19, emphasizing the need for preparedness in future respiratory pandemics. Universal access to advanced PPE, equitable resource distribution, and adaptive airway management strategies are critical components of a resilient healthcare system.

Additionally, ongoing research and innovation in non-invasive respiratory support and infection control will enhance the ability to manage high-risk patients effectively while protecting healthcare workers.

Key takeaways

☑ Level III PPE provides superior protection for healthcare workers during high-risk AGPs and should be prioritized.

☑ HFNO is a safe and effective respiratory support option when used with appropriate precautions.

☑ The timing of tracheal intubation should be individualized based on patient factors and response to non-invasive therapies.

☑ Harmonizing guidelines and ensuring global access to resources are essential for optimizing outcomes in airway management.

Additional recommended reading:

1. Wei H, Jiang B, Behringer EC, et al. Controversies in airway management of COVID-19 patients: updated information and international expert consensus recommendations. *Br J Anaesth.* 2021;126(2):361-366. PMID: 33256990; PMCID: PMC7836532.
2. Cook TM, El-Boghdadly K, McGuire B, et al. Consensus guidelines for managing the airway in patients with COVID-19. *Anaesthesia.* 2020;75(6):785-799. PMID: 32221970; PMCID: PMC7383579.
3. Rello J, Perez M, Roca O, et al. High-flow nasal therapy in adults with severe acute respiratory infection: a cohort study. *J Crit Care.* 2012;27(5):434-439. PMID: 22762937.

High-flow nasal oxygen, noninvasive ventilation, and conventional oxygen therapy in COVID-19 patients

17

Why this topic is important

The COVID-19 pandemic underscored the critical need for effective respiratory support strategies in managing acute respiratory failure (ARF). Invasive mechanical ventilation (IMV) has been the mainstay for severe cases but comes with significant risks, including ventilator-induced lung injury and ventilator-associated pneumonia. Noninvasive respiratory supports, such as high-flow nasal oxygen (HFNO), noninvasive ventilation (NIV), and conventional oxygen therapy (COT), offer less invasive alternatives that may prevent the need for IMV while reducing complications and resource burdens.

Despite widespread use, the comparative effectiveness of these noninvasive modalities in COVID-19 ARF remains to be seen. A recent systematic review and network meta-analysis by Pisciotta et al. 2024 provides critical insights into the relative benefits and risks of HFNO, NIV, and COT, aiming to guide clinicians in optimizing patient outcomes during pandemics and beyond.

Objectives of this update

- Compare HFNO, NIV, and COT in terms of treatment failure and mortality in patients with COVID-19-associated ARF.
- Highlight the potential advantages and limitations of each respiratory support modality.
- Provide evidence-based recommendations for selecting respiratory therapies in acute care settings.

What is new

- HFNO and NIV demonstrated comparable odds of treatment failure and mortality, with no significant differences relative to COT.
- Network meta-analysis ranked HFNO slightly higher in effectiveness but not statistically significantly better than NIV or COT.
- The findings emphasize the need for larger trials to refine understanding of the optimal use of noninvasive respiratory support in COVID-19 ARF.

Key findings

Study overview

The analysis included eight randomized controlled trials (RCTs) with 2,302 patients, stratified into three groups:

- HFNO: 1,175 patients (51%)
- NIV: 371 patients (16%)
- COT: 756 patients (33%)

The primary outcome was treatment failure, defined as discontinuation of the assigned therapy due to worsening disease. Mortality served as the secondary outcome.

Treatment failure

- HFNO and NIV showed comparable odds of treatment failure relative to COT.
- Pairwise comparisons between HFNO and NIV also revealed similar rates of treatment failure.

Mortality

- Mortality rates were consistent across HFNO, NIV, and COT groups.
- The probability of each modality ranking as the "best" for survival was almost equal: COT (34.7%), HFNO (33.7%), and NIV (31.6%).

Subgroup and sensitivity analyses

- Sensitivity analyses consistently suggested that HFNO might be advantageous in preventing treatment failure, although differences were not statistically significant.
- The consistency of findings across studies supports their reliability despite minor heterogeneity in patient characteristics and adjunctive therapies.

Recommendations for practice

Selecting a respiratory support strategy

1. High-flow nasal oxygen (HFNO):
HFNO may offer advantages in comfort and tolerance, particularly in patients with moderate-to-severe COVID-19 ARF who are not immediately at risk of progression to IMV.
Consider HFNO for settings where patient compliance and prolonged therapy are priorities.
2. Noninvasive ventilation (NIV):
NIV, including continuous positive airway pressure (CPAP), can be beneficial for patients requiring higher levels of pressure support to improve oxygenation and reduce breathing work.
Avoid routine use of NIV in patients with high risks of aerosol generation without adequate infection control measures.
3. Conventional oxygen therapy (COT):
COT remains an accessible option and may suffice for patients with mild ARF who do not demonstrate signs of rapid deterioration.
Reserve advanced modalities like HFNO and NIV for patients with more significant oxygenation deficits or increased respiratory effort.

Implementation considerations

- Monitoring and escalation: Closely monitor patients on HFNO or NIV for signs of treatment failure (e.g., escalating oxygen needs, persistent hypoxemia), ensuring timely transition to IMV when required.
- Resource availability: Align modality choice with available resources, including HFNO devices, ventilators, and healthcare personnel trained in noninvasive techniques.
- Infection control: Employ enhanced precautions, particularly with HFNO and NIV, to minimize aerosolization risks in high-transmission environments.

Broader implications

The findings highlight that HFNO and NIV are comparable to COT regarding treatment failure and mortality for COVID-19 ARF. These results contradict prior data in non-COVID ARF, where HFNO and NIV were associated with lower intubation and mortality rates. The study underscores the need for individualized patient care and suggests that in COVID-19, adjunctive therapies, disease-specific factors, and resource availability may play significant roles in determining outcomes.

Future research should focus on:

- Evaluating the long-term effects of noninvasive respiratory supports on recovery and quality of life.
- To optimize efficacy, explore combination strategies (e.g., alternating HFNO and NIV).
- Addressing specific patient subgroups, such as those with comorbidities or delayed presentation, to refine therapeutic guidelines.

Key takeaways

☑ HFNO, NIV, and COT showed no significant differences in treatment failure or mortality for COVID-19 ARF, emphasizing individualized care.

☑ HFNO may offer slight advantages in comfort and tolerance, while NIV provides higher pressure support for severe cases.

☑ Routine implementation should prioritize patient-specific needs, available resources, and infection control measures to optimize outcomes.

☑ Future trials are essential to refine the role of these modalities in pandemic and non-pandemic ARF management.

Additional recommended reading:

1. Pisciotta W, Passannante A, Arina P, et al. High-flow nasal oxygen versus conventional oxygen therapy and noninvasive ventilation in COVID-19 respiratory failure: a systematic review and network meta-analysis of randomized controlled trials. *Br J Anaesth.* 2024;132(5):936-944. PMID: 38307776; PMCID: PMC11103093.

2. Frat J-P, Quenot J-P, Badie J, et al. Effect of high-flow nasal cannula oxygen vs standard oxygen therapy on mortality in patients with respiratory failure due to COVID-19. *JAMA.* 2022;328(12):1212-1222. PMID: 36166027; PMCID: PMC9516287.

3. Grieco DL, Menga LS, Cesarano M, et al. Effect of helmet NIV vs HFNO on respiratory support in COVID-19: The HENIVOT trial. *JAMA.* 2021;325(17):1731-1743. PMID: 33764378; PMCID: PMC7995134.

Advances and techniques in airway management

Videolaryngoscopy for first-line intubation

18

Why this topic is important

Tracheal intubation is a critical component of airway management during surgical and emergency care. While most intubations proceed without incident, difficulty in airway management is associated with life-threatening complications, including hypoxia, aspiration, cardiovascular instability, and even death. Traditional Macintosh direct laryngoscopy (DL) has been the standard of care for decades, but it requires aligning airway axes for direct visualization of the glottis-a task that becomes increasingly challenging in patients with anatomical variations or limited mobility.

Videolaryngoscopy (VL) has emerged as a game-changing technology, using video cameras to enhance glottic visualization and reduce reliance on direct line-of-sight alignment. Despite its clear advantages, VL has predominantly been reserved for rescue situations after failed DL or in patients with anticipated difficult airways. The recent push to establish VL as a first-intention device challenges this paradigm, suggesting it could improve patient outcomes across the board.

Objectives of this update

- Review evidence supporting the use of VL as a first-line tool for tracheal intubation.
- Highlight procedural improvements and patient safety outcomes linked to VL implementation.
- Provide insights into overcoming barriers and promoting the adoption of VL in clinical settings.

What is new

Recent large-scale observational studies, including a 2022 publication by De Jong et al., provide compelling evidence that VL as a first-intention device improves intubation success rates and operator experience while reducing complications. The findings challenge long-standing practices and suggest VL may benefit all intubations, regardless of anticipated difficulty.

Practical insights into the use of videolaryngoscopy

Study design and outcomes

A quality improvement project conducted in two French teaching hospitals from March 2017 to September 2020 evaluated the impact of implementing VL as the first-choice device for tracheal intubation. One hospital adopted VL universally (compliant hospital), while the other retained its conventional practices (non-compliant hospital). The study encompassed over 26,000 intubations, divided into three phases: pre-intervention, implementation, and post-intervention.

Key findings include:

- **Improved ease of intubation:** The compliant hospital reported an increase in easy airway management from 94.3% pre-intervention to 98.7% post-intervention-a statistically significant improvement. In contrast, no significant changes were observed in the non-compliant hospital.
- **Reduced reliance on rescue techniques:** Post-intervention, the need for rescue intubation techniques dropped from 5.3% to 1.9% in the compliant hospital.
- **Enhanced operator experience:** Self-reported difficulty decreased significantly, reflecting the intuitive advantages of VL.

Structured implementation

The transition to VL as a first-line device was facilitated through a carefully designed implementation strategy:

- **Education and training:** All operators underwent training on VL devices, starting with manikins before advancing to patients. The training emphasized proper positioning, use of stylets, and managing initial learning curves.
- **Standardization:** The McGrath Mac video-laryngoscope was selected for its familiar design, resembling the traditional Macintosh laryngoscope, which minimized resistance and facilitated the adoption.
- **Supportive culture:** A team of airway experts provided ongoing guidance, addressed concerns, and encouraged consistent use of VL during the implementation phase.

The success of these measures highlights the importance of institutional commitment, user training, and clear communication in driving clinical change.

Why videolaryngoscopy works

1. **Enhanced visualization:** VL provides an indirect view of the glottis via a video feed, bypassing anatomical obstacles and enabling a better field of vision even in challenging cases.
2. **Increased success rates:** Improved visualization reduces the time to intubation and the number of failed attempts, minimizing patient risk.
3. **Reduced complications:** Studies consistently report fewer complications such as hypoxemia, esophageal intubation, and airway trauma with VL compared to DL.
4. **Safety during pandemics:** VL allows the operator to maintain a safer distance from the patient's airway, reducing the risk of infectious exposure.

Barriers to adoption

Despite its advantages, VL adoption as a universal first-intention technique faces several challenges:

- **Perceived loss of traditional skills:** Operators worry that widespread use of VL may erode expertise in DL, which is still essential in some situations, such as equipment failure.
- **Costs:** VL devices and their disposable blades are more expensive than traditional laryngoscopes, raising concerns about economic feasibility.
- **Resistance to change:** Transitioning from DL to VL represents a cultural shift that requires addressing entrenched practices and skepticism.

Overcoming challenges

The successful implementation of VL requires:

1. **Comprehensive training:** Addressing the learning curve and integrating VL into routine practice through hands-on sessions and simulation training.
2. **Cost-benefit analysis:** Emphasizing the long-term benefits of reduced complications, fewer adverse events, and enhanced safety.
3. **Integration with traditional techniques:** Ensuring continued training in DL alongside VL to preserve competence in both methods.

Clinical implications and the way forward

The findings from De Jong et al.'s study provide strong support for adopting VL as a first-line technique for tracheal intubation. The benefits are clear: higher success rates, reduced operator difficulty, and lower complication rates. These outcomes align with broader trends in airway management, including calls from experts and professional societies to make VL more accessible and widely used.

The implementation of VL also represents an opportunity to enhance training, improve patient safety, and adapt airway management practices to meet contemporary challenges, including infectious disease outbreaks. However, achieving universal adoption will require addressing financial and cultural barriers through institutional support, cost analysis, and continuous education.

Key takeaways

- ☑ Videolaryngoscopy significantly improves the ease and success of tracheal intubation compared to traditional direct laryngoscopy.
- ☑ A structured implementation strategy, including education, device standardization, and ongoing support, is key to successful adoption.
- ☑ Barriers such as cost and resistance to change can be addressed through training, communication, and highlighting VL's long-term benefits.
- ☑ The benefits of VL extend beyond anticipated difficult airways, supporting its use in all tracheal intubations.

Additional recommended reading:

1. De Jong A, Sfara T, Pouzeratte Y, et al. Videolaryngoscopy as a first-intention technique for tracheal intubation in unselected surgical patients: a before and after observational study. *Br J Anaesth.* 2022;129(4):624-634. PMID: 35811139.

2. Cook TM, Kelly FE. A national survey of videolaryngoscopy in the United Kingdom. *Br J Anaesth.* 2017;118:593-600. PMID: 28403414.

3. Apfelbaum JL, Hagberg CA, Connis RT, et al. 2022 American Society of Anesthesiologists practice guidelines for management of the difficult airway. *Anesthesiology.* 2022;136:31-81. PMID: 34762729.

Videolaryngoscopy or direct laryngoscopy for intubation

19

Why this topic is important

Tracheal intubation is a critical skill in anesthesia, critical care, and emergency medicine. Traditionally performed using direct laryngoscopy (DL), this procedure can be challenging, particularly in patients with difficult airways. Failed intubation is associated with significant risks, including hypoxemia, aspiration, cardiac arrest, and death. Videolaryngoscopy (VL), which uses video technology to enhance glottic visualization, has emerged as an alternative with the potential to improve success rates and patient safety.

Despite VL's advantages, its adoption has been inconsistent, hindered by cost considerations, lack of familiarity, and debates about its superiority in routine and emergency situations. A comprehensive Cochrane review by Hansel et al. 2022 synthesizes evidence from 222 randomized controlled trials (RCTs) involving over 26,000 participants. The review highlights VL's clear advantages over DL, providing robust evidence to guide its integration into routine practice.

Objectives of this update

- Highlight the comparative effectiveness of VL versus DL in adult patients.
- Explore specific advantages of different VL designs-Macintosh-style, hyperangulated, and channeled-and their clinical applications.
- Provide actionable recommendations for integrating VL into clinical practice.

What is new

Hansel et al.'s review, the largest of its kind, builds on earlier findings and introduces new evidence regarding VL's benefits across diverse clinical scenarios:

- VL reduces failed intubation rates by 56% and significantly improves first-pass success rates compared to DL.
- Hyperangulated VL demonstrates the greatest advantage in patients with difficult airways, reducing failed intubation rates by 71%.
- Evidence shows VL reduces hypoxemia and esophageal intubation rates while providing superior glottic visualization.
- Importantly, the review distinguishes between different VL designs, providing nuanced insights into their relative performance.

Comparative effectiveness of VL and DL

Overall benefits of VL

1. **Failed intubations:**
   - VL reduces the likelihood of failed intubations by 56% across all settings.
   - The advantage is particularly pronounced in patients with difficult airways, where VL reduces failed intubation rates by 71%.
2. **First-pass success:**
   - First-pass success is a critical metric in airway management, as multiple attempts increase the risk of complications such as hypoxemia and airway trauma.
   - VL improves first-pass success rates by 5% overall.
3. **Improved glottic views:**
   - VL decreases the proportion of poor laryngoscopic views (Cormack-Lehane grade 3 or 4) compared to DL. Hyperangulated VL designs provide the greatest improvement.

Patient safety outcomes

1. **Hypoxemia:**
   - Hypoxemia, defined as oxygen saturation < 94%, occurred 39% less frequently in VL cases across 41 studies. This is particularly significant in critically ill patients, where prolonged hypoxia can have severe consequences.
2. **Esophageal intubation:**
   - Esophageal intubation, a serious complication, was 61% less likely with hyperangulated VL than DL.
3. **Dental trauma:**
   - The incidence of dental injuries was not significantly different between VL and DL, though the evidence is of low certainty. Further studies are needed to clarify this risk.

VL designs: Macintosh-style, hyperangulated, and channeled

The review distinguishes between different VL designs, each with unique advantages.

Macintosh-style VL

- Retains the familiar shape of traditional DL blades but incorporates video imaging.
- Advantages:
  - 59% reduction in failed intubations.
  - 3% higher first-pass success compared to DL.
- Best suited for transitioning clinicians who are comfortable with DL but seek improved visualization.

Hyperangulated VL

- Features a sharply curved blade designed to visualize the glottis in patients with anterior airways.
- Advantages:
  - 71% reduction in failed intubations for difficult airways.
  - Lower rates of esophageal intubation.
- Requires pre-shaped stylets for optimal placement of the endotracheal tube (ETT), adding a layer of complexity.
- Ideal for managing anticipated or known difficult airways, including obese patients or those with restricted neck mobility.

Channeled VL

- Integrates a guiding channel to assist in ETT placement, simplifying the procedure.
- Advantages:
  - 57% reduction in failed intubations.
  - Easier to use for novice operators.
- Particularly useful in emergency scenarios or during rapid sequence induction (RSI).

Practical recommendations for VL implementation

Selecting the right VL device

- **Routine use:** Macintosh-style VL is ideal for elective surgeries where intubation is expected to be straightforward.
- **Difficult airways:** Hyperangulated VL should be prioritized for patients with anterior airways, obesity, or limited neck extension.
- **Training environments:** Channeled VL can accelerate learning for novices, providing a simpler intubation pathway.

Integrating VL into clinical workflows

1. **Operating rooms:**
    - Given its superior first-pass success and safety profile, VL should be the default device for routine and emergency intubations.
2. **ICUs and emergency departments:**
    - Critically ill patients or those in emergency settings benefit most from VL, where rapid desaturation makes first-pass success imperative.

Clinician training

- Structured training is essential to maximize VL's effectiveness:
    - Begin with hands-on sessions using both manikins and patients.
    - Emphasize the importance of blade selection, stylet shaping, and handling hyperangulated devices.
    - Incorporate VL training into airway management courses and credentialing requirements.

Cost considerations

- While VL devices involve higher upfront costs, the reduction in complications (e.g., failed intubation, hypoxemia, esophageal intubation) can offset these expenses over time.
- Hospitals should assess the cost-effectiveness of transitioning to VL as the primary intubation method.

Challenges

1. **Learning curve:**
    - Operators accustomed to DL may require time and training to adapt to VL techniques, particularly hyperangulated designs.
2. **Device availability:**
    - Resource-limited settings may face challenges in acquiring and maintaining VL devices.

Clinical implications and the way forward

This review provides compelling evidence that VL offers superior outcomes to DL, particularly in patients with difficult airways. The advantages of VL are clear across metrics such as first-pass success, failed intubation rates, and hypoxemia prevention. Widespread adoption of VL, coupled with structured training and device standardization, can revolutionize airway management, improving safety and efficiency in diverse clinical settings.

Key takeaways

☑ Videolaryngoscopy significantly reduces failed intubation rates, particularly in patients with difficult airways.

☑ Hyperangulated VL provides the greatest benefit in terms of visualization and esophageal intubation prevention, though it requires familiarity with pre-shaped stylets.

☑ Training programs and institutional protocols should prioritize the integration of VL into routine and emergency airway management.

☑ Cost-effectiveness analyses support VL's use as the first-line intubation tool, given its ability to reduce complications.

Additional recommended reading:

1. Hansel J, Rogers AM, Lewis SR, et al. Videolaryngoscopy versus direct laryngoscopy for adults undergoing tracheal intubation: a Cochrane systematic review and meta-analysis update. *Br J Anaesth.* 2022;129(4):612-623. PMID: 35820934; PMCID: PMC9575044.

2. Woodall NM, Cook TM. National census of airway management techniques used for anaesthesia in the UK: first phase of the Fourth National Audit Project at the Royal College of Anaesthetists. *Br J Anaesth.* 2011;106(2):266-271. PMID: 21131655.

3. Adams JP, Murphy PG. Obesity in anaesthesia and intensive care. *Br J Anaesth.* 2000;85(1):91-108. PMID: 10927998.

Airway management in critically ill patients with videolaryngoscopy

20

Why this topic is important

Tracheal intubation in critically ill patients is one of the most challenging procedures in medicine, with a high potential for complications such as cardiovascular instability, hypoxemia, and esophageal intubation. The stakes are especially high in emergency settings, where patients often present with compromised physiology and complex anatomy, leaving little margin for error.

First-pass success during intubation is critical to minimizing these risks, as multiple attempts increase the likelihood of adverse events, including cardiac arrest and severe hypoxemia. While videolaryngoscopy has become increasingly popular in emergency and critical care settings, its efficacy and safety profile compared to traditional direct laryngoscopy remain subjects of an ongoing investigation.

Russotto et al. (2023) provide a comprehensive analysis of video laryngoscopy's performance in critically ill patients as part of the INTUBE study, a large international cohort study. Their findings highlight video laryngoscopy's benefits in improving first-pass success and reducing specific complications, offering a robust basis for integrating this technology into routine critical care practice.

Objectives of this update

- Evaluate the benefits of videolaryngoscopy over direct laryngoscopy in critically ill patients.
- Analyze the risks and adverse event profiles associated with videolaryngoscopy.
- Provide evidence-based recommendations for optimizing its use in critical care.

What is new

- Videolaryngoscopy increased first-pass intubation success by 40% compared to direct laryngoscopy.
- Patients with videolaryngoscopy experienced fewer esophageal intubations.
- No significant increase in major adverse events, including hypoxemia or cardiovascular instability, was associated with videolaryngoscopy.

Key findings

Improved first-pass success

- Videolaryngoscopy achieved first-pass success in 84% of cases, compared to 79% with direct laryngoscopy.
- The device was particularly beneficial for patients with predictors of difficult intubation, such as high Mallampati scores, limited cervical spine mobility, or obesity.
- Video laryngoscopy provides improved glottic visualization, reducing the need for excessive cervical spine manipulation and facilitating safer intubation in anatomically challenging cases.

Reduced esophageal intubation

- Esophageal intubation occurred significantly less frequently with videolaryngoscopy (16.2%) than with direct laryngoscopy.
- This advantage is critical in critical care settings, where esophageal intubation can be life-threatening and often goes unrecognized due to limited capnography use.

Safety profile

- Despite concerns about prolonged laryngoscopy attempts, videolaryngoscopy was not associated with higher rates of major peri-intubation adverse events, such as cardiovascular collapse or severe hypoxemia.
- Cardiac arrest occurred less frequently with videolaryngoscopy (1.6%) than with direct laryngoscopy, suggesting a potential protective effect in physiologically fragile patients.

Implications for clinical practice

Patient selection and preparation

- Patient characteristics: Videolaryngoscopy should be the preferred method for patients with predictors of difficult intubation, including obesity, cervical spine immobilization, and high Mallampati scores.
- Pre-intubation optimization: Adequate preoxygenation, hemodynamic stabilization, and airway assessment are essential to maximize the safety and effectiveness of intubation.

Training and proficiency

- Operator expertise plays a significant role in video laryngoscopy outcomes. Studies suggest that a minimum of 20-30 intubations with the device is necessary to achieve proficiency.
- Regular simulation-based training and deliberate practice should be integrated into airway management curricula for critical care providers to enhance skills and confidence.

Device selection and resource allocation

- Device options: Modern video laryngoscopes, including hyperangulated and Macintosh-type blades, should be available to accommodate a range of anatomical challenges. Hyperangulated blades may be especially useful for patients with limited mouth openings or anterior airways.
- Adjuncts: Backup devices and adjuncts, such as bougies, stylets, and supraglottic airway devices, are critical for successful intubation with videolaryngoscopy.
- Availability: Ensuring that video laryngoscopes are widely available in ICUs and emergency departments is essential for standardizing high-quality airway management across healthcare settings.

Protocols and guidelines

- Implementing standardized airway ma-nagement protocols that prioritize videolaryngoscopy for high-risk patients can enhance the first-pass success and reduce variability in clinical outcomes.
- Protocols should include pre-intubation checklists, algorithms for failed intubation, and strategies for managing peri-intubation adverse events.

Broader implications

The findings from Russotto et al. (2023) reinforce the importance of video laryngoscopy as a primary airway management tool in critical care. By improving first-pass success and reducing complications such as esophageal intubation, video laryngoscopy has the potential to significantly enhance patient safety and outcomes in high-stakes environments.

Future research should address:

- Long-term outcomes associated with videolaryngoscopy in critically ill patients, including its impact on ICU mortality and recovery.
- Cost-effectiveness analyses to determine the feasibility of widespread implementation in resource-constrained settings.
- The role of emerging technologies, such as artificial intelligence-guided airway management systems, in further improving the safety and efficiency of videolaryngoscopy.

Additionally, the integration of videolaryngoscopy into global airway management guidelines will require collaboration among anesthesiologists, critical care specialists, and emergency medicine professionals to ensure consistent application and training.

Key takeaways

☑ Videolaryngoscopy increases first-pass intubation success by 40% compared to direct laryngoscopy, particularly in patients with difficult airway predictors.

☑ The device significantly reduces esophageal intubation rates, enhancing patient safety during high-risk intubations.

☑ Major peri-intubation adverse events, such as cardiovascular collapse and hypoxemia, are not increased with videolaryngoscopy, supporting its safety profile.

☑ Widespread adoption of videolaryngoscopy in emergency and ICU settings requires systematic training, resource allocation, and standardized protocols.

Additional recommended reading:

1. Russotto V, Lascarrou JB, Tassistro E, et al. Efficacy and adverse events profile of videolaryngoscopy in critically ill patients: subanalysis of the INTUBE study. *Br J Anaesth*. 2023;131(3):607-616. PMID: 37208282.
2. Cook TM, El-Boghdadly K, McGuire B, et al. Consensus guidelines for managing the airway in patients with COVID-19: a move towards universal videolaryngoscopy. *Anaesthesia*. 2020;75(6):785-99. PMID: 32221970; PMCID: PMC7383579.
3. Higgs A, McGrath BA, Goddard C, et al. Guidelines for tracheal intubation in critically ill adults. *Br J Anaesth*. 2018;120(2):323-352. PMID: 29406182.

Artificial intelligence and imaging in difficult airway management

21

Why this topic is important

Managing a difficult airway remains one of the most critical and complex challenges in anesthesia and intensive care. Errors in identifying or addressing difficult airways can lead to significant complications, including hypoxia, trauma, and cardiac arrest. Traditional methods of difficult airway assessment rely on clinical scores such as Mallampati classification or thyromental distance, but their sensitivity and specificity leave much to be desired.

Artificial intelligence (AI) offers a transformative potential in this field. Both machine learning (ML) and deep learning (DL), subsets of AI, have shown significant promise. ML involves identifying patterns in data to make predictions. At the same time, DL is a specialized form of ML that processes complex imaging data to identify features and classify outcomes with exceptional accuracy. DL models, in particular, leverage large datasets, combining imaging and clinical information to deliver accurate predictions and real-time guidance. AI-enhanced approaches promise to revolutionize how clinicians evaluate and manage airways, ensuring greater precision, efficiency, and safety.

Objectives of this update

- Summarize advancements in AI and imaging techniques for airway management.
- Highlight AI's role in predicting and managing difficult airways using various imaging modalities.
- Discuss the clinical implications of integrating AI into routine practice.

What is new

Recent developments in AI and DL have introduced predictive models capable of identifying difficult airways with higher sensitivity and specificity than traditional methods. These models integrate imaging techniques-such as X-ray, CT, MRI, and facial recognition-with clinical parameters to generate comprehensive and personalized assessments. Additionally, intelligent intubation devices utilizing real-time feedback are on the horizon, potentially reshaping airway management.

Practical insights into AI applications in airway management

Current AI tools and their applications

AI models are increasingly applied to airway management, utilizing both imaging and clinical data to predict difficult airways. De Rosa et al.'s 2024 review outlines the primary AI tools, including:

- **Machine learning (ML):** Identifies patterns in imaging and clinical data to predict airway challenges.
- **Deep learning (DL):** Processes complex imaging data for segmentation and classification tasks, such as identifying airway anatomy or predicting difficult laryngoscopy.
- **Artificial neural networks (ANNs):** Analyzes features like vocal fold positioning from endoscopic images.
- **Big data analytics:** Combines clinical records with imaging to develop robust predictive algorithms.

Imaging techniques integrated with AI

1. **X-ray-based AI models:**
    - X-ray imaging is widely accessible and used for visualizing airway structures.
    - DL models improve accuracy in detecting malpositioned endotracheal tubes (ETTs) and predicting difficult laryngoscopy. For example, AI-enhanced X-rays can evaluate parameters like thyromental distance and neck circumference to identify anatomical challenges.
2. **Computed tomography (CT):**
    - CT scans provide detailed 3D reconstructions of airway anatomy, helping clinicians assess airway volume, length, and structural abnormalities.
    - Machine-learning algorithms trained on CT data predict challenges such as obstructive airway disorders or nasal intubation difficulties, achieving predictive values exceeding 90% in some studies.
3. **Magnetic resonance imaging (MRI):**
    - While less frequently used due to high costs and prolonged imaging times, MRIs offer superior visualization of soft tissue structures.
    - AI applied to MRI data can analyze features like tongue positioning and airway obstruction, aiding in personalized airway management plans.
4. **Facial imaging:**
    - AI models trained on facial photographs have shown promise in predicting difficult airways by analyzing morphological traits. For instance, a model using frontal and lateral images achieved an area under the receiver operating characteristic curve (AUROC) of 0.864, demonstrating high sensitivity and specificity.

Intelligent intubation devices

Intelligent intubation devices equipped with AI algorithms are emerging as powerful tools in airway management. These devices include:

- **Video laryngoscopes:** Enhanced with DL models for automated detection of anatomical landmarks, these tools provide real-time feedback during intubation.
- **Wearable sensors:** Monitor resistance and pressure changes to guide the operator, reducing the risk of esophageal intubation or trauma.
- **Automated endoscopy systems:** Accurately identify airway structures and potential obstructions, assisting clinicians during complex cases.

Limitations and challenges

Despite the promise of AI in airway management, several challenges remain:

1. **Data quality and bias:**
    - Many AI models are trained on datasets that may not represent diverse populations, limiting generalizability.
    - Variability in clinical practices and imaging techniques can affect model accuracy.
2. **Integration into clinical practice:**
    - Real-world application of AI tools requires seamless integration with existing workflows, including electronic health record systems.
    - Training and acceptance among clinicians are essential for widespread adoption.
3. **Cost and accessibility:**
    - High costs of advanced imaging modalities and AI systems may restrict their use in resource-rich settings.

Key takeaways

☑ AI models utilizing imaging and clinical data are transforming difficult airway management, offering superior predictive accuracy compared to traditional methods.

☑ Integrating AI with X-ray, CT, MRI, and facial imaging enhances the ability to assess airway challenges and guide interventions.

☑ Intelligent intubation devices provide real-time feedback, reducing complications and improving success rates.

☑ Challenges include data bias, cost, and the need for clinician training, but ongoing advancements promise widespread clinical adoption.

Additional recommended reading:

1. De Rosa S, Bignami E, Bellini V, Battaglini D. The Future of Artificial Intelligence Using Images and Clinical Assessment for Difficult Airway Management. *Anesth Analg.* 2024 Apr 1. PMID: 38557728.
2. Zhou C-M, Wang Y, Xue Q, et al. Predicting difficult airway intubation in thyroid surgery using multiple machine learning and deep learning algorithms. *Front Public Health.* 2022;10:937471. PMID: 36033770; PMCID: PMC9399522.
3. Hayasaka T, Kawano K, Kurihara K, et al. Creation of an artificial intelligence model for intubation difficulty classification by deep learning using face images: An observational study. *J Intensive Care.* 2021;9:38. PMID: 33952341; PMCID: PMC8101256.
4. Naik NB, Mathew PJ, Kundra P. Scope of artificial intelligence in airway management. *Indian J Anaesth.* 2024;68(1):105-110. PMID: 38406331; PMCID: PMC10893795.

Ultrasound in airway management

22

Why this topic is important

Ultrasound has revolutionized multiple areas of clinical practice, and its application in airway management is no exception. By providing real-time imaging of airway structures, ultrasound can enhance the accuracy of critical procedures such as endotracheal intubation, cricothyroidotomy, and airway assessment. Unlike traditional techniques that rely heavily on physical examination or indirect visualization, ultrasound offers noninvasive, radiation-free, and cost-effective solutions, improving outcomes across diverse patient populations.

Despite its potential, the adoption of airway ultrasound remains variable. A structured understanding of its applications-from identifying challenging airways to guiding therapeutic interventions-is crucial for integrating this technology into routine clinical practice.

Objectives of this update

- Highlight key applications of ultrasound in airway management, including its role in predicting difficult intubation and confirming endotracheal tube (ETT) placement.
- Provide evidence-based insights into the use of ultrasound for emergency airway access.
- Outline practical steps for incorporating ultrasound into clinical practice.

What is new

Ultrasound-guided airway management is gaining recognition for its versatility. Key advancements discussed in a recent article by Gomes et al. include:

- Sonographic measurements are used to predict difficult laryngoscopy with high sensitivity and specificity.
- Improved techniques for real-time confirmation of endotracheal tube placement, avoiding complications such as esophageal intubation.
- Development of the TACA (thyroid cartilage-airline-cricoid cartilage-airline) approach for accurate localization of the cricothyroid membrane during emergency front-of-neck access.

Practical applications of airway ultrasound

Predicting difficult laryngoscopy

Ultrasound provides quantitative tools to predict airway difficulty. Examples include:

1. **Skin-to-hyoid distance:**
   - A distance > 1.28 cm predicts difficult laryngoscopy with 85% sensitivity and specificity.
2. **Skin-to-epiglottis distance:**
   - A distance > 2.5 cm suggests potential difficulty, with a female-specific sensitivity of 100% and specificity of 83%.
3. **Hyomental distance ratio (HMDR):**
   - Calculated as the hyomental distance in an extended position divided by that in a neutral position. An HMDR ≤ 1.2 predicts difficult laryngoscopy with 100% sensitivity and 90.5% specificity.
4. **Tongue thickness and volume:**
   - Measurements > 6.1 cm or volumes > 121 cm^3 are associated with difficult intubation.

These parameters allow for preemptive planning, such as preparing advanced airway tools (e.g., videolaryngoscopes or fiberoptic scopes).

Confirming endotracheal intubation

Ultrasound can confirm ETT placement with real-time imaging:

- **Technique:**
  - Place a linear probe transversely at the suprasternal notch to visualize the trachea and esophagus simultaneously.
  - Correct tracheal placement is indicated by hyperechoic lines of the ETT visible within the anterior tracheal lumen.
  - Esophageal intubation creates a "double trachea" sign, identifying the ETT in the esophagus.
- **Advantages:**
  - Reduces reliance on auscultation or chest X-ray.
  - It avoids delays in detecting esophageal intubation, improving patient safety.

Guiding emergency front-of-neck access

Front-of-neck access, such as cricothyrotomy, is a high-risk procedure, especially in patients with indistinct anatomy. Ultrasound can improve success rates:

- **TACA approach:**
  - The thyroid cartilage-airline-cricoid cartilage-airline (TACA) approach involves locating the cricothyroid membrane with a linear probe.
  - The cricothyroid membrane is marked on the skin using ultrasound before initiating the procedure.
- **String-of-pearls sign:**
  - In the sagittal plane, the tracheal rings appear as oval structures resembling pearls. This image helps center the cricothyroid membrane for accurate access.

Sizing endotracheal tubes

In pediatric patients, where airway size is critical, ultrasound provides an effective method to determine the optimal ETT size:

- Place a linear probe at the cricoid cartilage level and measure the transverse diameter of the air column.
- Select an ETT with an outer diameter slightly smaller than the measured air column to minimize airway trauma.

Integrating ultrasound into practice

Training and proficiency

1. **Education:**
    - Basic ultrasound training should include airway sonoanatomy, image acquisition techniques, and interpretation of key findings.
2. **Simulation:**
    - Hands-on practice using high-fidelity simulators or cadavers enhances skill acquisition and confidence.
3. **Competency assessment:**
    - Periodic evaluations ensure clinicians maintain proficiency in both technical and interpretive aspects.

Workflow integration

1. **Pre-procedural planning:**
    - Use ultrasound to identify at-risk patients and prepare advanced airway tools or techniques.
2. **Emergency readiness:**
    - Incorporate portable ultrasound machines into airway carts for rapid deployment during emergencies.
3. **Standardized protocols:**
    - Develop institutional guidelines for ultrasound use in airway assessment and interventions.

Challenges

- **Equipment availability:** Portable ultrasound machines may not be accessible in resource-limited settings.
- **Learning curve:** Achieving proficiency requires time and practice.
- **Standardization:** Variability in techniques and parameters across studies complicates widespread adoption.

Key takeaways

☑ Ultrasound enhances airway management by improving the prediction of difficult intubation, guiding emergency access, and confirming ETT placement.

☑ Key parameters such as skin-to-hyoid distance, HMDR, and tongue volume offer reliable metrics for predicting challenging airways.

☑ The TACA approach and "double trachea" sign improve the accuracy of life-saving interventions such as cricothyrotomy.

☑ Widespread implementation requires standardized protocols, hands-on training, and integration into airway management workflows.

Additional recommended reading:

1. Gomes SH, Canelli R, Corradi F, et al. The use of ultrasound in airway management. *Anesth Analg.* 2024;139(4):887-890. PMID: 39284139.
2. Kristensen MS. Ultrasonography in the management of the airway. *Acta Anaesthesiol Scand.* 2011;55(9):1155-1173. PMID: 22092121.
3. Rai Y, You-Ten E, Siddiqui N. The role of ultrasound in front-of-neck access for cricothyroid membrane identification: a systematic review. *J Crit Care.* 2020;60:161-168. PMID: 32836091.

Point-of-care ultrasound (POCUS) in emergency airway management

23

Why this topic is important

Emergency airway management outside the operating room (OR) is a high-stakes procedure associated with significant morbidity and mortality. Critically ill patients undergoing tracheal intubation (TI) often face complications such as cardiovascular collapse, hypoxemia, and cardiac arrest, with peri-intubation hemodynamic instability occurring in nearly 43% of cases. These risks are exacerbated by limited diagnostic information and the challenges of managing physiologically compromised patients.

Point-of-care ultrasound (POCUS) is emerging as a critical tool in this context. Its ability to provide real-time insights into respiratory, cardiac, and vascular status makes it invaluable for optimizing patient care before, during, and after airway management. By tailoring interventions to individual physiological needs, POCUS has the potential to mitigate complications and improve outcomes in patients with physiologically difficult airways (PDA). In addition, POCUS supports a more comprehensive approach to airway management by enhancing situational awareness and reducing reliance on guesswork, particularly in emergencies.

Objectives of this update

- Review the role of POCUS in identifying and managing physiologically difficult airways, ensuring its effective application in diverse emergency scenarios.
- Discuss its utility in pre-intubation planning, such as hemodynamic optimization, hypoxemia evaluation, and aspiration risk assessment, to reduce procedural complications.
- Provide actionable recommendations for integrating POCUS into emergency airway workflows, fostering better decision-making and improved patient safety.

What is new

- POCUS enhances the identification of high-risk airway conditions, such as pericardial effusion, pneumothorax, and hypovolemia, enabling targeted interventions.
- Lung ultrasound and focused cardiac assessment protocols have been refined to support pre-intubation preparation and decision-making.
- Algorithms integrating POCUS into airway management workflows offer structured guidance for emergency scenarios.

Key findings

Physiologically difficult airway

POCUS is instrumental in managing PDAs by addressing the physiological perturbations predisposing patients to TI complications. Hypoxemia, hypotension, and elevated intracranial pressure are common contributors to airway challenges.

1. Hypoxemia
   - Lung ultrasound can identify underlying causes such as pneumothorax, atelectasis, or acute respiratory distress syndrome (ARDS).
   - Findings from lung ultrasound can guide strategies like preoxygenation with noninvasive ventilation (NIV) or high-flow nasal oxygen, ensuring optimized alveolar recruitment.
2. Hypotension
   - Rapid ultrasound in shock (RUSH) protocols can evaluate cardiac contractility, right ventricular strain, and inferior vena cava (IVC) collapsibility to guide fluid resuscitation or vasopressor therapy.
   - In cases of tamponade physiology, POCUS can identify pericardial effusion, necessitating tailored induction strategies to maintain hemodynamic stability.
3. Aspiration risk
   - Gastric ultrasound can quantify gastric volume, identifying patients at high risk of aspiration. This information supports decisions regarding rapid sequence induction (RSI) or awake intubation.

Optimizing intubation with POCUS

POCUS provides dynamic feedback during intubation to enhance safety and efficacy:

- Screening for anatomical difficulty: Ultrasound can visualize structures like the cricothyroid membrane, aiding in the preparation for potential surgical airways.
- Confirming endotracheal tube (ETT) placement: Bilateral lung sliding and real-time visualization of the ETT cuff prevent complications like mainstem intubation or esophageal placement.

Recommendations for practice

Pre-intubation assessment

1. Lung ultrasound:
   - Use protocols like BLUE (bedside lung ultrasound in emergency) to evaluate lung aeration, detect pneumothorax, and guide preoxygenation strategies.
2. Cardiac assessment:
   - Perform focused echocardiography to identify cardiac tamponade, reduced ventricular contractility, or hyperdynamic states requiring inotropic support or fluid resuscitation.
3. Gastric evaluation:
   - Antral cross-sectional area (ACSA) measurements assess aspiration risk, particularly in non-fasting or critically ill patients.

During intubation

- Ensure real-time confirmation of ETT placement using ultrasound to detect bilateral lung sliding and exclude esophageal intubation.

Post-intubation optimization

- Reassess hemodynamic parameters and lung aeration to address complications such as tension pneumothorax or worsening pulmonary edema.

Broader implications

Integrating POCUS into emergency airway management represents a paradigm shift in care. Enabling rapid, accurate, and non-invasive assessments enhances the safety and precision of interventions. Widespread adoption of POCUS can improve outcomes by reducing peri-intubation complications and tailoring care to individual patient needs. In resource-limited settings, the availability of portable and handheld POCUS devices further broadens its applicability, offering critical support where advanced imaging modalities may not be accessible.

Future priorities include:

- Developing standardized training programs to ensure competency in POCUS use among clinicians.
- Conducting large-scale studies to validate POCUS protocols in diverse clinical settings.
- Leveraging advancements in handheld ultrasound technology to increase accessibility and usability.

Key takeaways

☑ POCUS is a game-changing tool for managing physiologically difficult airways in emergency settings, improving decision-making and procedural safety.

☑ It enables targeted interventions by identifying conditions like hypoxemia, hypotension, and aspiration risk, effectively addressing individual patient needs.

☑ Structured algorithms integrating POCUS into airway workflows reduce complications and enhance team coordination in high-stakes scenarios.

☑ Training, standardization of protocols, and innovations in ultrasound technology are critical for enabling widespread and equitable adoption.

Additional recommended reading:

1. Khorsand S, Chin J, Rice J, et al. Role of point-of-care ultrasound in emergency airway management outside the operating room. *Anesth Analg.* 2023;137:124-136. PMID: 36693019.
2. Mosier JM, Sakles JC, Whitmore SP, et al. The physiologically difficult airway: A concept to optimize patient safety. *West J Emerg Med.* 2015;16:1109-1117.PMID: 26759664; PMCID: PMC4703154.
3. Austin DR, Chang MG, Bittner EA. Handheld point-of-care ultrasound in emergency airway management. *Chest.* 2021;159:1155-1165. PMID: 32971075.

Videolaryngoscopy or direct laryngoscopy for airway management in pediatric anesthesia

24

Why this topic is important

Effective airway management is a cornerstone of pediatric anesthesia, as failed intubation can result in severe complications, including hypoxia, airway trauma, and cardiovascular instability. The choice of laryngoscopy technique-direct laryngoscopy (DL) or videolaryngoscopy (VL)-is critical in ensuring patient safety and procedural success.

Videolaryngoscopy, with its improved visualization of the glottis via a camera at the blade's tip, has been widely advocated for managing difficult airways. However, its role in elective pediatric intubation must be clarified, particularly in patients without predicted airway difficulties. A recent randomized controlled trial (RCT) by Klabusayova et al. (2021) provides valuable insights by comparing VL and DL for elective airway management in children, exploring success rates, intubation times, and complication rates.

Objectives of this update

- Review evidence comparing VL and DL for elective intubation in pediatric patients with normal airways.
- Discuss the advantages and challenges of VL in routine pediatric airway management.
- Recommend selecting the appropriate laryngoscopy technique based on patient needs and procedural goals.

What is new

- VL demonstrated better glottic visualization (Cormack-Lehane grade 1 views) but did not outperform DL regarding first-attempt success rates.
- Despite its enhanced visualization capabilities, VL was associated with longer intubation times compared to DL.
- Both techniques achieved 100% overall intubation success, with no significant differences in complication rates between the two groups.

Key findings

Study design and outcomes

The study included 501 pediatric patients undergoing elective surgery. Patients were randomized to either the VL or DL group. The primary outcome was the first-attempt intubation success rate, while secondary outcomes included intubation time, overall success, and complications (e.g., desaturation, bradycardia).

1. First-attempt success rates:
    - DL outperformed VL, with success rates of 92.6% versus 86.8%.
    - The difference was attributed to VL's steeper learning curve and operator dependency, as even improved glottic visualization did not translate to higher success rates.
2. Intubation time:
    - The mean time for successful intubation was significantly longer for VL (39.0 ± 36.7 seconds) compared to DL (23.6 ± 24.7 seconds).
3. Glottic visualization:
    - VL provided superior glottic views, with 83.1% achieving Cormack-Lehane grade 1 visualization compared to 68.0% in the DL group.
4. Complications:
    - Both groups had similar low rates of adverse events, including desaturation (< 5%), bradycardia (< 1%), and no incidents of aspiration or traumatic intubation.

Factors influencing VL performance

- Operator experience: Success rates for VL were slightly lower among less experienced practitioners, highlighting the need for adequate training in VL techniques.
- Blade design: Differences in blade types (e.g., Macintosh vs. Miller) and operator preferences may have contributed to variability in VL outcomes.

Recommendations for practice

Choosing between VL and DL

1. Patient factors:
    - VL is recommended for anticipated difficult airways due to its superior glottic visualization.
    - DL remains an efficient and reliable choice for routine intubation in patients with normal airways.
2. Operator expertise:
    - Adequate training in VL is essential to maximize its potential benefits and minimize longer intubation times.
    - Simulation-based training can help anesthesiologists build proficiency in VL techniques.
3. Clinical context:
    - VL is particularly beneficial in settings requiring airway documentation or when team-based visualization of the airway is advantageous.

Optimizing VL outcomes

- Practice and preparation: Regular use of VL in elective cases can enhance operator familiarity and reduce intubation times.
- Blade selection: Choose the appropriate blade design and size based on patient age and anatomical considerations.

Broader implications

This study underscores the need for a nuanced approach to airway management in pediatric anesthesia. While VL offers clear advantages in glottic visualization, its routine use in elective intubation may not always confer superior outcomes compared to DL.

Further research should explore:

- The impact of structured VL training on intubation success and efficiency.
- Patient-specific factors that predict better outcomes with VL versus DL.
- Cost-effectiveness analyses to guide equipment allocation and decision-making in resource-limited settings.

Key takeaways

☑ Direct laryngoscopy achieved higher first-attempt success rates and faster intubation times than videolaryngoscopy in elective pediatric airway management.

☑ Videolaryngoscopy provided superior glottic visualization but required more time for successful intubation, emphasizing the importance of operator skill.

☑ Both techniques were equally safe, with no significant differences in complication rates.

☑ Videolaryngoscopy remains an invaluable tool for difficult airways and should be incorporated into training and practice to ensure readiness for challenging cases.

Additional recommended reading:

1. Klabusayova E, Klucka J, Kosinova M, et al. Videolaryngoscopy vs. direct laryngoscopy for elective airway management in paediatric anaesthesia: A prospective randomised controlled trial. *Eur J Anaesthesiol.* 2021;38(10):1187-1193. PMID: 34560686.
2. Aziz MF, Dillman D, Brambrink AM. Comparative effectiveness of video laryngoscopy in the setting of predicted difficult airway. *Anesthesiology.* 2012;116(3):629-636. PMID: 22261795.
3. Hu X, Jin Y, Li J, et al. Efficacy and safety of videolaryngoscopy versus direct laryngoscopy in pediatric intubation: A meta-analysis of 27 randomised trials. *J Clin Anesth.* 2020;66:109968. PMID: 32645564.

Airway management in emergency and critical situations

Videolaryngoscopy or direct laryngoscopy for emergency intubation

25

Why this topic is important

Emergency endotracheal intubation (EEI) is a critical procedure for securing the airway in life-threatening situations, such as severe trauma, cardiac arrest, or respiratory failure. Compared to planned intubations in controlled environments, EEI poses significant challenges, including time constraints, patient instability, and limited resources. These factors contribute to lower first-attempt success rates and higher complication risks, such as aspiration, hypoxia, and airway injuries.

Direct laryngoscopy (DL) has traditionally been the standard endotracheal intubation technique. However, advancements in video laryngoscopy (VL) have revolutionized airway management by offering enhanced visualization of the vocal cords and minimizing cervical spine manipulation. Despite the potential benefits, VL's effectiveness compared to DL in emergency settings has remained unclear, with prior studies producing mixed results. A systematic review and meta-analysis by Alsabri et al. (2024) synthesizes data from 14 randomized controlled trials (RCTs) to provide definitive insights into VL's role in improving EEI outcomes.

Objectives of this update

- To evaluate the comparative effectiveness of video and direct laryngoscopy in achieving first-attempt and overall intubation success rates.
- To assess the impact of VL on intubation-related complications, procedure time, and visualization quality.
- To highlight key implications for clinical practice and areas for future research.

What is new

This review by Alsabri et al. 2024 consolidates evidence from 14 RCTs involving 2,470 patients to evaluate VL versus DL in emergency intubation. The key findings reveal:

- VL significantly improves the first-attempt success rate compared to DL.
- VL reduces upper airway injuries and esophageal intubations.
- VL enhances visualization quality, as measured by the percentage of glottis opening (POGO) scores.
- No significant difference exists in overall intubation success rates between VL and DL.

Key findings

First-attempt success rate

VL demonstrated a statistically significant advantage over DL for first-attempt intubation success. This finding highlights VL's potential to reduce the risks of repeated intubation attempts, such as hypoxia and hemodynamic instability.

Intubation difficulty score and visualization

VL reduced the mean intubation difficulty score (IDS) by 0.62 points compared to DL, reflecting its ease of use and efficiency. Additionally, VL improved peri-intubation POGO scores by 24.91 percentage points, offering superior glottic visualization. These advantages are particularly valuable in anatomically challenging airways or scenarios requiring rapid intervention.

Safety and complications

VL was associated with lower rates of upper airway injuries and esophageal intubation. Although VL reduced the risk of aspiration, this finding did not reach statistical significance. Other complications, including desaturation and cardiac arrest, showed no significant differences between the two techniques.

Intubation time

The analysis showed that VL reduced first-attempt intubation time by an average of 6.92 seconds compared to DL. However, the two groups had no significant difference in overall intubation time.

Advantages of video laryngoscopy

1. Improved first-attempt success: VL enhances visualization and eliminates the need for strict alignment of the airway axes, making it especially advantageous in patients with difficult anatomy.
2. Enhanced safety profile: Lower rates of complications, such as esophageal intubation and airway trauma, contribute to better patient outcomes.
3. Reduced provider fatigue: VL's ergonomic design and superior visualization can ease procedural stress, particularly in prolonged or challenging cases.

Challenges and limitations

1. Heterogeneity among studies: Variability in VL devices, patient populations, and clinical settings limits the generalizability of findings.
2. Operator expertise: Successful use of VL requires adequate training and experience, which may not be universally available.
3. Cost considerations: VL devices are more expensive than traditional DL, potentially limiting access in resource-constrained settings.

Implications for practice

The findings support integrating VL as the first-choice modality for emergency intubations, particularly in high-risk patients or scenarios where first-attempt success is critical. However, widespread implementation requires investment in training programs and equitable access to VL devices.

Recommendations for future research

1. Device comparisons: Future studies should evaluate differences among various VL systems to identify the most effective models for emergency use.
2. Pediatric populations: There is a need for dedicated research on the efficacy of VL in children, who often present unique anatomical and physiological challenges.
3. Long-term outcomes: Further investigation is needed to assess whether improved first-attempt success rates translate into better survival and functional outcomes.

Key takeaways

- ☑ VL offers significant advantages over DL in first-attempt intubation success, safety, and visualization quality during emergency airway management.
- ☑ The reduced complication rates with VL, such as fewer airway injuries and esophageal intubations, highlight its value in critical settings.
- ☑ Adequate training and resource allocation are essential to maximize the benefits of VL.
- ☑ While VL improves first-attempt success rates, overall intubation success rates are comparable between VL and DL, suggesting DL remains a viable alternative when VL is unavailable.

Additional recommended reading:

1. Alsabri M, Abdelwahab OA, Elsnhory AB, et al. Video laryngoscopy versus direct laryngoscopy in achieving successful emergency endotracheal intubations: A systematic review and meta-analysis. *Systematic Reviews*. 2024;13:85. PMID: 38475918; PMCID: PMC10935931.
2. Brown CA, Kaji AH, Fantegrossi A, et al. Video laryngoscopy compared to augmented direct laryngoscopy in adult emergency department tracheal intubations. *Acad Emerg Med*. 2020;27:100. PMID: 31957174.
3. Cook TM, Woodall N, Frerk C. Fourth National Audit Project: Major complications of airway management in the UK. *Br J Anaesth*. 2011;106:617-631. PMID: 21447488.

Delayed or rapid sequence intubation (RSI) in trauma patients

26

Why this topic is important

Trauma patients often present with critical injuries necessitating urgent airway management, where rapid sequence intubation (RSI) is the standard approach to achieve rapid airway control while minimizing the risk of aspiration. RSI involves administering an intravenous anesthetic, applying cricoid pressure once the lash reflex is lost, and promptly placing an endotracheal tube (ETT). This approach is prioritized in patients with preserved airway reflexes. However, in obtunded or arrested patients, intubation is typically performed without medications.

Despite its efficiency, RSI can predispose critically injured patients to peri-intubation hypoxia, particularly when preoxygenation is suboptimal. Hypoxia during intubation is a significant concern as it can exacerbate secondary injuries, worsen hemodynamic instability, and lead to poor outcomes, including brain injury progression.

In contrast, delayed sequence intubation (DSI) has emerged as an alternative strategy, particularly in patients requiring more definitive assessment and stabilization before intubation. DSI focuses on optimizing oxygenation through sedative-assisted preoxygenation, delaying paralysis and intubation until oxygenation is improved. By incorporating noninvasive oxygenation techniques, DSI aims to minimize peri-intubation hypoxia, which is particularly critical in trauma patients to prevent further exacerbation of brain and systemic injuries.

A study by Bandyopadhyay et al. (2023) compared the incidence of peri-intubation hypoxia between RSI and DSI in trauma patients, offering valuable insights into their relative effectiveness and safety. While RSI remains the cornerstone for airway management in emergency scenarios, this study highlights DSI as a potential alternative in select trauma patients, where improved preoxygenation could mitigate hypoxia and optimize outcomes.

Objectives of this update

- To evaluate the incidence of peri-intubation hypoxia in trauma patients undergoing DSI versus RSI.
- To explore the hemodynamic and procedural implications of DSI in critically injured patients.
- To provide recommendations for the adoption and optimization of DSI in trauma settings.

What is new

This retrospective cohort study by Bandyopadhyay et al. 2023 analyzed trauma registry data to compare DSI and RSI outcomes in trauma triage.

Key findings include:

- Lower incidence of peri-intubation hypoxia in the DSI group compared to RSI.
- Comparable intubation success rates and first-pass success between groups.
- Improved preoxygenation efficacy in DSI, with more patients achieving SpO_2 > 94% prior to intubation.
- No significant differences in post-intubation complications, including aspiration and cardiac arrest.
- While DSI requires more time to intubate, this delay is offset by improved oxygen reserves and reduced desaturation risk.

Key findings

Study design and population

- Design: Retrospective cohort study using trauma registry data.
- Participants: Adult trauma patients (aged ≥18 years) requiring emergency intubation on arrival to trauma triage.
- Intervention groups:
  - RSI group: Paralysis and intubation performed without sedative-assisted preoxygenation.
  - DSI group: Sedation was administered to facilitate preoxygenation before paralysis and intubation.
- Outcomes
  - Primary: Incidence of peri-intubation hypoxia (SpO_2 < 90%).
  - Secondary: Intubation success rates, first-pass success, time to intubation, and post-intubation complications.

Results

1. Peri-intubation hypoxia:
   - DSI significantly reduced the incidence of peri-intubation hypoxia compared to RSI.
2. Intubation success:
   - Comparable success rates and first-pass success between RSI and DSI.
3. Preoxygenation efficacy:
   - DSI achieved SpO_2 > 94% before intubation in a significantly higher proportion of patients.
4. Time to intubation:
   - DSI required more time to intubate but reduced the risk of desaturation.
5. Complications:
   - Post-intubation aspiration and cardiac arrest rates were similar between RSI and DSI groups.

Clinical implications

Benefits of DSI

- Avoid unnecessary intubation in patients who may stabilize with noninvasive ventilation.
- Allows time to address life-threatening issues before proceeding with intubation.
- Improves pre-intubation oxygenation, particularly in patients at high risk of desaturation during RSI.

Challenges of DSI

- Airway compromise: Risk increases if the patient's condition deteriorates during preoxygenation.
- Monitoring: Respiratory failure may occur if the patient is not closely observed.
- Rapid intubation: Clinicians must be prepared to perform emergent intubation if the situation changes.

Balancing time and safety

While DSI introduces a slight delay, its ability to improve oxygen reserves justifies its use in trauma patients prone to rapid desaturation.

Recommendations

1. **Adopt DSI in trauma triage:**
   - Integrate DSI protocols for patients at risk of desaturation during RSI.
2. **Training trauma teams:**
   - Educate teams to identify DSI candidates and practice sedation-assisted preoxygenation techniques.
3. **Personalized approach:**
   - Tailor the choice of intubation technique based on:
     - Patient condition
     - Severity of trauma
     - Feasibility of preoxygenation
   - Ensure equipment readiness: functioning suction, various ETT sizes, laryngoscopes, capnography, and wide-bore cannulas for rapid anesthetic delivery.

Sedative choices

- Propofol: Ideal for hemodynamically stable patients but not suitable for frail or hypovolemic patients.
- Ketamine: Effective in hypovolemic or prehospital settings; increases BP and HR but requires antisialagogues (e.g., glycopyrrolate).
- Etomidate: Safe in hemodynamic instability but contraindicated in adrenal suppression and limited in availability.
- Thiopentone: Rapid action with minimal hemodynamic effects; however, extravasation and intra-arterial injection are hazardous.
- Midazolam: Useful in obtunded patients.

Neuromuscular blockers

- Succinylcholine: Rapid onset but associated with myalgia, hyperkalemia, and increased intraocular/intracranial tension.
- Rocuronium: A safer alternative with similar efficacy.

Limitations and future directions

1. Study limitations:
   - Retrospective design limits the ability to control for confounding factors.
   - Single-center data may not be generalized to other trauma systems.
   - Lack of long-term outcome data, such as survival or functional recovery, restricts assessing DSI's overall impact.
2. Future research:
   - Prospective trials to compare DSI and RSI in diverse trauma populations.
   - Investigations into the optimal sedative agents and doses for preoxygenation.
   - Studies assess the cost-effectiveness and logistical feasibility of DSI in high-volume trauma centers.

Key takeaways

☑ DSI significantly reduces peri-intubation hypoxia without compromising intubation success.

☑ It is particularly beneficial for trauma patients at high risk of desaturation during RSI.

☑ A tailored, patient-specific approach, proper training, and equipment readiness are essential for successful implementation.

Additional recommended reading:

1. Bandyopadhyay S, Al-Kawaz MN, Lazarus HM, et al. Peri-intubation hypoxia after delayed sequence intubation versus rapid sequence intubation in critically injured patients on arrival to trauma triage: A retrospective cohort study. *Anesth Analg*. 2023;137(1):140-149. PMID: 37058727.

2. Weingart SD, Trueger NS, Wong N, et al. Delayed sequence intubation: A novel approach to emergent airway management in the agitated patient. *Ann Emerg Med*. 2015;65(4):424-430. PMID: 25447559.

3. Janz DR, Semler MW, Lentz RJ, et al. Randomized trial of apneic oxygenation during endotracheal intubation of critically ill patients. *Am J Respir Crit Care Med*. 2016;193(3):273-280. PMID: 26426458; PMCID: PMC4803060.

Factors influencing first-pass intubation in prehospital RSI

27

Why this topic is important

First-pass success (FPS) in rapid sequence intubation (RSI) is a critical determinant of patient outcomes during prehospital emergency airway management. Each additional intubation attempt significantly increases the risk of complications, such as hypoxemia, aspiration, airway trauma, and cardiac arrest. The variability of FPS rates in prehospital settings, ranging from 59% to 98%, reflects the challenges of intubating patients in unpredictable and resource-limited environments.

Understanding the factors influencing FPS can guide improvements in clinical practice, equipment choices, and operator training. Hayes-Bradley et al. (2024) conducted a systematic review and meta-analysis to identify predictive and protective factors for FPS, offering evidence-based insights into improving airway management outcomes in prehospital settings.

Objectives of this update

- Identify key predictive factors associated with failed first-pass intubation in prehospital RSI.
- Highlight protective strategies and techniques that enhance FPS.
- Provide actionable recommendations for clinicians and services to optimize prehospital airway management.

What is new

The review by Hayes-Bradley et al. synthesizes evidence from 97 studies covering over 26,000 prehospital intubations. Key findings include:

- Blood or fluid in the airway, limited mouth opening, and restricted neck movement are significant predictors of failed FPS.
- Protective factors include experienced operators, videolaryngoscopy (VL) with bougies, and patient positioning strategies like head-up tilt.
- Training and simulation for prehospital providers remain essential for improving FPS rates.

Predictive factors for failed first-pass success

Patient-related factors

1. **Airway contamination:**
   - Blood, vomitus, or secretions in the airway significantly reduce visualization, impeding FPS.
2. **Anatomical challenges:**
   - Restricted neck mobility, limited mouth opening, and craniofacial abnormalities are strongly associated with difficult intubations.
3. **Trauma-related factors:**
   - Facial injuries, burns, and cervical spine precautions increase intubation difficulty.
   - Trauma patients have a higher rate of failed FPS than medical patients.
4. **Extremes of age:**
   - Infants (< 1 year) are particularly at risk due to small airway size and rapid desaturation.

Environmental factors

1. **Nighttime operations:**
   - Reduced visibility and fatigue contribute to lower FPS rates during night missions.
2. **On-ground intubation:**
   - Performing intubation at ground level increases difficulty compared to stretcher-based procedures.

Protective factors for improving FPS

Equipment and techniques

1. **Videolaryngoscopy with bougies:**
   - VL improves glottic visualization, while bougies assist in difficult tube placements.
   - VL with bougies significantly increases FPS rates, particularly in anatomically challenging cases.
2. **Patient positioning:**
   - Elevating the head or placing the patient in a head-up tilt enhances oxygenation and airway alignment.
3. **Suction and airway clearance:**
   - Effective suctioning reduces airway contamination, facilitating successful intubation.

Operator-related factors

1. **Experience and training:**
   - FPS rates are higher with experienced intubators, including anesthetists and critical care providers.
   - Regular training and simulation improve technical skills and non-technical skills like teamwork and decision-making.
2. **Team dynamics:**
   - Effective communication and role clarity within the intubation team enhance success rates.

Actionable recommendations for clinicians

Pre-intubation preparation

1. **Comprehensive airway assessment:**
   - Evaluate for predictive factors, such as blood in the airway or anatomical challenges.
   - Anticipate the need for advanced equipment and techniques.
2. **Optimize patient positioning:**
   - Use stretcher-based, head-up positioning to improve airway alignment and reduce contamination risks.
3. **Ensure equipment readiness:**
   - Always have videolaryngoscopes, bougies, and suction devices available for prehospital intubations.

During intubation

1. **Use VL for challenging airways:**
   - Hyperangulated VL is especially effective in managing anterior larynxes or restricted views.
2. **Employ suction early and often:**
   - Clear blood, vomitus, or secretions to maintain visibility.
3. **Limit intubation attempts:**
   - Adopt a maximum of two attempts per provider before escalating to alternative techniques, such as supraglottic airway devices (SGAs).

Training and education

1. **Simulation-based training:**
   - Include high-fidelity scenarios that replicate prehospital challenges, such as trauma, limited visibility, and adverse environments.
2. **Focused feedback:**
   - Provide constructive reviews of intubation attempts to identify areas for improvement.

Implications for practice and research

Addressing heterogeneity

The study emphasizes the variability in prehospital RSI practices, highlighting the need for standardized protocols to reduce disparities in FPS rates. Further research should focus on:

1. **Comparative studies of VL designs:**
   - Evaluate the performance of different VL devices in various prehospital scenarios.
2. **Impact of environmental factors:**
   - Assess strategies for mitigating nighttime and on-ground challenges.

Technology and innovation

Emerging technologies, such as artificial intelligence-assisted laryngoscopy and enhanced imaging systems, hold promise for improving FPS rates in prehospital settings.

Key takeaways

☑ Predictive factors for failed FPS include blood in the airway, anatomical challenges, and nighttime intubations.

☑ Protective strategies, such as videolaryngoscopy with bougies, head-up positioning, and operator experience, significantly improve FPS rates.

☑ To optimize outcomes, prehospital services should prioritize equipment readiness, simulation-based training, and adherence to standardized protocols.

Additional recommended reading:

1. Hayes-Bradley C, McCreery M, Delorenzo A, et al. Predictive and protective factors for failing first-pass intubation in prehospital rapid sequence intubation: an aetiology and risk systematic review with meta-analysis. *Br J Anaesth.* 2024;132(5):918-935. PMID: 38508943.
2. Walker PW, Burdette M, Susi L, Guyette FX, Martin-Gill C. Association between First-pass Intubation Success and Enhanced PPE Use during the COVID-19 Pandemic. Prehosp Emerg Care. 2024;28(2):209-214. PMID: 36780396.
3. Miller M, Storey H, Andrew J, Christian E, Hayes-Bradley C. Out-of-Hospital Pediatric Video Laryngoscopy With an Adult Device: A Case Series Presented With a Contemporary Group Intubated With Direct Laryngoscopy. Pediatr Emerg Care. 2023;39(9):666-671. PMID: 36790879.

Tracheal intubation in critically ill patients with difficult airways

28

Why this topic is important

Tracheal intubation in critically ill adults is a high-risk procedure, frequently associated with significant complications. When anatomical challenges combine with physiological derangements such as hypoxemia, hemodynamic instability, or intracranial hypertension, the airway is classified as a physiologically difficult airway (PDA). These patients are particularly vulnerable to peri-intubation hypoxemia, cardiovascular collapse, and increased mortality. Such complications underscore the need for meticulous preparation and evidence-based strategies to optimize outcomes.

Managing a PDA requires more than technical skill-it demands a deep understanding of pathophysiology, precise procedural techniques, and a coordinated team approach. A recent Delphi study by Karamchandani et al. provides consensus-based recommendations to address the challenges of PDA management in critically ill adults, offering actionable strategies to enhance patient safety.

Objectives of this update

- Define the physiologically difficult airway and identify its associated risks.
- Summarize expert consensus on preparation, procedural techniques, and hemodynamic optimization.
- Provide practical recommendations to improve outcomes in PDA management.

What is new

The Delphi consensus highlights:

- Routine preoxygenation using noninvasive ventilation (NIV) or high-flow nasal oxygen (HFNO) as the standard for improving oxygen reserves in hypoxemic patients.
- Modified rapid sequence intubation (RSI) techniques, emphasizing hemodynamic stability through tailored induction agents and early vasopressor use.
- First-line use of videolaryngoscopy (VL) for improved visualization and higher first-pass success rates in physiologically challenging scenarios.

Defining the physiologically difficult airway

A PDA arises from severe pathophysiological abnormalities that complicate airway management, even when anatomy is favorable. Its defining features include:

1. **Hypoxemia:**
   - Present in conditions such as acute respiratory distress syndrome (ARDS) or cardiogenic shock, hypoxemia shortens the safe apnea time, leading to rapid desaturation during intubation.
2. **Cardiovascular instability:**
   - Hemodynamic collapse can result from induction agents, the transition to positive-pressure ventilation, or sympathetic withdrawal.
3. **Right ventricular (RV) dysfunction:**
   - RV failure exacerbates hemodynamic instability, particularly in pulmonary hypertension or large pulmonary embolism.
4. **Intracranial hypertension:**
   - Elevated intracranial pressure (ICP) in conditions like traumatic brain injury demands meticulous control to avoid further increases that could precipitate herniation.

Patients with obesity or pregnancy also demonstrate PDA characteristics due to reduced functional residual capacity (FRC) and higher oxygen consumption.

Preparing for tracheal intubation in PDAs

Structured preparation and team dynamics

1. **Checklists and team communication:**
   - Use a structured checklist to verify equipment, drugs, and backup strategies.
   - Conduct a pre-intubation briefing to ensure clarity of roles, particularly in high-stakes settings.
2. **Airway assessment:**
   - Combine anatomical assessments (e.g., Mallampati, neck mobility) with tools like the MACOCHA score to anticipate both anatomical and physiological challenges.

Oxygenation strategies

1. **Preoxygenation:**
   - NIV and HFNO are preferred methods for improving oxygen reserves:
     - NIV optimizes alveolar recruitment in patients with severe hypoxemia (PaO_2/FiO_2 ratio < 200).
     - HFNO provides apneic oxygenation, extending the safe apnea window.
   - Position patients in the head-elevated laryngoscopy position (HELP) to enhance oxygenation and prevent aspiration.
2. **Apneic oxygenation:**
   - Use nasal cannula at 10-15 L/min during apnea to maintain oxygenation during intubation.

Procedural strategies for managing PDAs

Induction and intubation

1. **Rapid sequence intubation (RSI):**
   - A modified RSI approach is favored for PDAs to balance hemodynamic stability and aspiration prevention:
     - Induction agents:
       - Use ketamine or etomidate instead of propofol for their favorable hemodynamic profiles.
       - Avoid high-dose sedatives that exacerbate hypotension.

- Neuromuscular blockade:
    - Administer neuromuscular blocking agents (NMBAs) like rocuronium or succinylcholine to ensure optimal intubation conditions.
- Mask ventilation:
    - Gentle ventilation may be necessary to prevent desaturation in severely hypoxemic patients.

2. **Videolaryngoscopy (VL):**
    - VL is the first-line tool for intubation in PDAs, offering superior visualization and higher first-pass success rates than direct laryngoscopy.
    - Use hyperangulated blades for anteriorly positioned larynges.
3. **Adjuncts:**
    - Use a stylet or bougie to facilitate tube placement, particularly in challenging cases.

Managing hemodynamics during intubation

Preventing cardiovascular collapse

1. **Pre-induction hemodynamic optimization:**
    - Administer vasopressors (e.g., norepinephrine) prophylactically to stabilize blood pressure during induction.
    - Assess fluid responsiveness using point-of-care ultrasound (POCUS) or passive leg raising, but avoid indiscriminate fluid boluses.
2. **Post-intubation strategies:**
    - Transition patients to lung-protective ventilation settings:
        - Low tidal volumes (6-8 mL/kg predicted body weight).
        - Moderate positive end-expiratory pressure (PEEP ≥5 cmH_2O) to prevent alveolar collapse.

Post-intubation care

1. **Confirm tube placement:**
    - Use waveform capnography as the gold standard to verify endotracheal placement.
2. **Control ventilation and oxygenation:**
    - Monitor for ventilator-induced compli-cations such as barotrauma or volutrauma, particularly in ARDS patients.
3. **Manage sedation and ICP:**
    - Maintain adequate sedation to prevent agitation and further increases in ICP in patients with intracranial hypertension.

Improving team readiness

Simulation-based training

- Regular simulation exercises replicate physiologically difficult airway scenarios, enhancing both technical skills (e.g., VL use) and non-technical skills like communication and role allocation.

Role clarity

- Assign specific roles to team members (e.g., intubation lead, drug administration, backup ventilation) to streamline workflows and minimize errors.

Key takeaways

- ☑ The physiologically difficult airway (PDA) is defined by hypoxemia, cardiovascular instability, and other pathophysiological risks, requiring careful planning and execution.
- ☑ Preoxygenation with NIV or HFNO and apneic oxygenation strategies are critical for improving oxygen reserves and extending the safe apnea window.
- ☑ Modified rapid sequence intubation with tailored induction agents, early vasopressors, and videolaryngoscopy optimizes safety and success.
- ☑ Post-intubation care, including lung-protective ventilation and sedation management, is essential for preventing secondary complications.
- ☑ Simulation training and structured team protocols are crucial for preparing clinicians to manage these high-risk scenarios effectively.

Additional recommended reading:

1. Karamchandani K, Nasa P, Jarzebowski M, et al. Tracheal intubation in critically ill adults with a physiologically difficult airway: an international Delphi study. Intensive Care Med. 2024;50:1563—1579. PMID: 39162823.
2. Russotto V, Myatra SN, Laffey JG, et al. Intubation practices and adverse peri-intubation events in critically ill patients from 29 countries. JAMA. 2021;325:1164—1172. PMID: 33755076; PMCID: PMC7988368.
3. Higgs A, McGrath BA, Goddard C, et al. Guidelines for the management of tracheal intubation in critically ill adults. Br J Anaesth. 2018;120:323—352. PMID: 29406182.

Emergency airway management outside the OR

29

Why this topic is important

Airway management is a critical skill in anesthesiology, yet the complexity increases significantly when performed outside the operating room (OR). Locations such as the intensive care unit (ICU), emergency department (ED), or general wards present unique challenges that elevate the risk of complications. These include anatomical difficulties, physiologic instability, and logistical constraints, all of which can lead to life-threatening outcomes.

Recent studies highlight that peri-intubation complications, such as cardiovascular collapse and severe hypoxemia, occur in nearly half of all emergency airway interventions outside the OR. Despite advances in devices and techniques, adherence to best practices and standardized protocols remains inconsistent, further exacerbating poor outcomes. This update, based on the findings of Jarzebowski et al. (2022), explores the key challenges, outcomes, and strategies to optimize emergency airway management in non-OR settings.

Objectives of this update

- Identify the unique challenges of airway management outside the OR.
- Highlight the impact of peri-intubation adverse events on patient outcomes.
- Provide recommendations to improve safety and success in emergency airway interventions.

What is new

- Cardiovascular collapse is the most frequent adverse event during emergency intubation, occurring in 42.6% of cases.
- First-pass success remains critical for reducing complications but requires attention to physiologic optimization.
- New approaches, such as awake video laryngoscopy and physiologically informed strategies, are gaining attention for their potential to improve outcomes.

Key findings

Common challenges

1. Anatomic difficulties
    - Anatomical predictors of difficult airways (e.g., short neck, limited mouth opening) are prevalent, with 46.8% of patients having at least one predictor.
    - Emergent situations often limit time for thorough airway assessments, reducing the utility of predictive bedside tests.
2. Physiologic instability
    - Many critically ill patients present with reduced cardiovascular and respiratory reserves. Intubation-induced hypotension and hypoxemia are frequent and severe.
    - Positive pressure ventilation post-intubation exacerbates conditions like refractory hypoxemia and hemodynamic instability, leading to increased morbidity and mortality.
3. Logistical and situational barriers
    - Limited access to advanced airway equipment, vasopressors, and experienced personnel complicates interventions.
    - Space constraints and suboptimal patient positioning hinder effective intubation.

Outcomes of emergency airway management

- Peri-intubation adverse events: A major international study reported that at least one adverse event occurred in 45.2% of critically ill patients. Cardiovascular collapse (42.6%) and severe hypoxemia (9.3%) were the most common, while cardiac arrest occurred in 3.1%.
- Impact on mortality: These complications significantly increased ICU and 28-day mortality rates.
- Success metrics: First-pass success rates of 79.8% were achieved, but multiple attempts were associated with higher complication rates.

Strategies to improve outcomes

Physiologic optimization

- Preoxygenation: Utilize noninvasive positive-pressure ventilation or high-flow nasal oxygen to optimize oxygen reserves before intubation, particularly in hypoxic patients.
- Hemodynamic stabilization: Administer vasopressors and fluids judiciously to mitigate post-intubation hypotension. Emerging evidence suggests that pre-emptive vasopressor use may reduce cardiovascular collapse.
- Induction agents: Use hemodynamically stable agents like etomidate or low-dose ketamine to minimize sympathetic suppression during induction.

Enhancing first-pass success

- Device selection: Videolaryngoscopy improves first-pass success compared to direct laryngoscopy, especially in patients with predictors of difficult airways.
- Technique optimization: Head-elevated or ramped positioning can improve glottic visualization and intubation success.
- Skill and training: Regular simulation-based training for non-anesthesiology clinicians (e.g., emergency or ICU teams) ensures readiness for high-risk scenarios.

Logistical improvements

- Standardized protocols: Multiple studies have shown that implementing checklists and airway management bundles that include preoxygenation, fluid resuscitation, and equipment preparation has reduced adverse events.
- Access to resources: It is critical to ensure safe intubation that non-OR locations are equipped with essential tools, such as waveform capnography and advanced airway devices.

Broader implications

Emergency airway management outside the OR demands an integrated approach that addresses anatomical, physiological, and logistical challenges. Standardized protocols, along with the widespread availability of advanced airway equipment and pre-intubation optimization strategies, can significantly reduce complications.

Future research should prioritize:

- Developing physiologically informed guidelines for managing critically ill patients during intubation.
- Evaluating emerging technologies, such as automated facial analysis for predicting difficult airways and awake video laryngoscopy, to improve first-pass success.
- Expanding access to training programs in LMICs, where logistical and resource limitations further complicate emergency airway management.

Key takeaways

☑ Emergency airway management outside the OR is associated with high rates of peri-intubation complications, particularly cardiovascular collapse and severe hypoxemia.

☑ First-pass success is critical for minimizing complications and improving outcomes, with videolaryngoscopy playing a key role.

☑ Physiologic optimization, including preoxygenation and hemodynamic stabilization, is essential for safe and effective intubation.

☑ Standardized protocols and better resource allocation are necessary to overcome logistical challenges and ensure preparedness.

Additional recommended reading:

1. Jarzebowski M, Estime S, Russotto V, Karamchandani K. Challenges and outcomes in airway management outside the operating room. Curr Opin Anaesthesiol. 2022;35(2):109-114. PMID: 35102045
2. Russotto V, Myatra SN, Laffey JG, et al. Intubation practices and peri-intubation events in critically ill patients: results from the INTUBE study. JAMA. 2021;325(12):1164-1172. PMID: 33755076; PMCID: PMC7988368.
3. Higgs A, McGrath BA, Goddard C, et al. Guidelines for tracheal intubation in critically ill adults. Br J Anaesth. 2018;120(2):323-352. PMID: 29406182.

Strategies for emergency airway management outside the OR

30

Why this topic is important

Emergency airway management outside the operating room (OR) often involves critically ill patients with minimal physiological reserve, exposing them to higher risks of complications than elective cases. Locations like intensive care units (ICUs), emergency departments, and radiology suites frequently lack the optimal infrastructure, equipment, and staffing found in OR settings. These environments present unique challenges, blending anatomical, physiological, and situational difficulties, often leading to adverse events such as hypoxemia, cardiovascular collapse, or failed airway attempts.

With complication rates as high as 45% in emergent cases, it is imperative to adopt evidence-based strategies tailored to out-of-OR airway management. By addressing specific challenges and employing structured approaches, clinicians can mitigate risks and improve outcomes for this vulnerable patient population.

Objectives of this update

- Identify the specific challenges associated with out-of-OR airway management.
- Highlight effective strategies for preparation, patient optimization, and intubation techniques.
- Provide practical recommendations to enhance safety and efficacy in emergency airway scenarios.

What is new

Key updates on managing out-of-OR airways include:

- Integration of the PREPARE checklist (Preoxygenate, Resist distractions, Examine, Plan, Adjust, Review, Exit) to streamline preparation and execution.
- Evidence supporting high-flow nasal oxygenation (HFNO) and noninvasive ventilation (NIV) for superior preoxygenation and apneic oxygenation.
- Recognition of the importance of tailored patient positioning and hemodynamic optimization to minimize peri-intubation complications.

Understanding the unique challenges of out-of-OR airway management

Situational and logistical factors

Emergency airway management in non-OR environments often suffers from:

- **Limited infrastructure:** Poor access to the patient's head, inadequate lighting, and confined spaces can impede successful intubation.
- **Inadequate equipment:** Advanced airway devices like videolaryngoscopes (VL), fiber-optic bronchoscopes, and emergency invasive airway tools may be unavailable.
- **Personnel constraints:** Limited availability of trained providers and support staff during emergencies compounds the challenge.

Patient-specific factors

Patients requiring emergent airway interventions often present with the following:

- **Anatomically difficult airways:** Conditions like maxillofacial trauma, cervical spine injury, or airway masses complicate visualization and intubation.
- **Physiologically difficult airways:** Reduced functional residual capacity, ventilation-perfusion mismatches, and hemodynamic instability increase the risk of desaturation and cardiovascular collapse.

Evidence-based strategies for optimizing airway management

Preparation and assessment

1. **Structured pre-intubation checklists:**
   - The PREPARE checklist ensures compre-hensive preparation, focusing on preoxygenation, equipment readiness, and backup plans.
   - Team huddles to clarify roles and discuss contingencies improve communication and readiness.
2. **Airway assessment:**
   - Tools like the MACOCHA score (Mallampati, sleep Apnea, Cervical mobility, Opening of mouth < 3 cm, Coma, Hypoxemia, Anesthetist absence) predict risks by combining anatomical and physiological parameters.
   - Bedside evaluations (e.g., Mallampati classification) guide the choice of equipment and techniques.

Oxygenation techniques

1. **Preoxygenation:**
   - HFNO and NIV enhance oxygenation in patients with severe respiratory compromise, particularly those with high oxygen demands or intrapulmonary shunting.
   - NIV is particularly effective in patients with PaO_2/FiO_2 ratios < 200.
2. **Apneic oxygenation:**
   - A nasal cannula, delivering oxygen during apnea, extends safe intubation windows and prevents desaturation.

Patient positioning

- **Ramped position:** Elevating the torso aligns the airway axes, optimizing preoxygenation and reducing aspiration risk, especially in obese patients.
- **Sniffing position:** Ideal for improving glottic visualization in patients with limited neck mobility.

Intubation techniques

1. **Videolaryngoscopy:**
   - VL significantly increases first-pass success and reduces esophageal intubation rates compared to direct laryngoscopy (DL).
   - Hyperangulated blades are particularly beneficial for anteriorly positioned larynges

2. **Rapid sequence intubation (RSI):**
   - RSI minimizes aspiration risk by rapidly inducing unconsciousness and neuromuscular blockade.
   - Avoidance of manual ventilation between induction and intubation remains controversial; gentle ventilation may prevent desaturation in select cases.
3. **Delayed sequence intubation (DSI)**
   - While RSI prioritizes rapid intubation, DSI focuses on improving oxygenation in patients at risk of severe hypoxia before intubation.

Addressing hemodynamic instability

Peri-intubation hypotension occurs in up to 46% of critically ill patients, driven by the interplay of pharmacologic agents, positive-pressure ventilation, and reduced sympathetic drive.

Prevention strategies

1. **Fluid resuscitation:**
   - Pre-intubation fluid boluses are of limited benefit and may exacerbate hypoxemia in non-volume-responsive patients.
   - Passive leg raising or point-of-care ultrasound (POCUS) can identify candidates for fluid optimization.
2. **Vasopressors:**
   - Prophylactic administration of bolus or continuous vasopressors, such as norepinephrine, stabilizes hemodynamics during induction.

Improving team dynamics and training

1. **Crisis resource management (CRM):**
   - Emphasize situational awareness, closed-loop communication, and role clarity to prevent errors.
2. **Simulation-based training:**
   - Scenarios replicating high-risk, low-frequency emergencies prepare providers for real-world challenges.

Practical recommendations for clinicians

Pre-procedure

- Utilize the PREPARE checklist for thorough preparation.
- Ensure availability of advanced airway tools and backup devices, including VL and supraglottic airways.

During intubation

- Optimize patient positioning to facilitate visualization and oxygenation.
- Use VL as the first-line tool for anatomically challenging airways.
- Monitor hemodynamic parameters closely, intervening early with fluids or vasopressors.

Post-intubation

- Assess for complications such as hypotension, hypoxemia, or unrecognized esophageal intubation.
- Debrief with the team to identify areas for improvement.

Key takeaways

- ☑ Emergency airway management outside the OR involves unique challenges that require tailored approaches.
- ☑ Structured preparation, advanced oxygenation techniques, and VL improve success rates and reduce complications.
- ☑ Hemodynamic optimization with tailored fluid and vasopressor strategies is critical for peri-intubation safety.
- ☑ Training in CRM and simulation-based scenarios enhances team performance and patient outcomes.

Additional recommended reading:

1. Karamchandani K, Wheelwright J, Yang AL, et al. Emergency airway management outside the operating room: current evidence and management strategies. Anesth Analg. 2021;133(3):648-662. PMID: 34153007.
2. Cook TM, Woodall N, Harper J, et al. Major complications of airway management in the UK: results of the Fourth National Audit Project. Br J Anaesth. 2011;106:632-642. PMID: 21447489.
3. De Jong A, Molinari N, Rolle A, et al. Early identification of patients at risk for difficult intubation in the intensive care unit. Am J Respir Crit Care Med. 2013;187:832-839. PMID: 23348979.
4. Rebollar RE, Hierro PL, Fernández AMM. Delayed Sequence Intubation in Children, Why Not?. Saudi J Med Med Sci. 2024;12(2):117-124. PMID: 38764564; PMCID: PMC11098273.

Prehospital emergency front-of-neck airway techniques

31

Why this topic is important

Front-of-neck airway (FONA) is a critical, last-resort airway procedure performed when conventional airway securing methods fail. While rare in prehospital settings, its execution is often the difference between life and death. The technique is particularly vital in "cannot intubate, cannot oxygenate" (CICO) scenarios, where immediate action is required to restore ventilation and prevent catastrophic hypoxia.

Over the years, multiple approaches to FONA have been developed, including surgical and needle techniques. However, discrepancies in success rates and variations in training and equipment highlight the need for evidence-based guidelines. The 2017 UK prehospital guidelines promoted surgical FONA as the first-line method, emphasizing its higher success rates and greater reliability than needle techniques.

Objectives of this update

- Summarize the findings of a systematic review and meta-analysis by Morton et al. (2023) on prehospital FONA success rates.
- Compare the effectiveness of surgical versus needle-based techniques in achieving successful airway access.
- Provide practical recommendations for optimizing FONA implementation in diverse clinical and prehospital settings.

What is new

- The study revealed an overall FONA success rate of 88% across various settings, with surgical techniques achieving the highest median success rate of 100%.
- Since the 2017 UK guidelines, surgical FONA techniques have been increasingly adopted, with a slight improvement in success rates compared to prior years.
- Pediatric FONA data remain limited, necessitating further research to identify optimal techniques for younger patients.

Key findings

Comparative success rates

The systematic review analyzed 69 studies encompassing 3,292 FONA attempts, with 1,229 cases included in the meta-analysis. Key findings include:

- Surgical techniques: The pooled success rate was 92%, with a median of 100%.
- Needle techniques: Pooled success rates were significantly lower at 52%, with a median of 50%.
- Tracheostomy kits: These achieved a pooled success rate of 87%, highlighting outcome variability based on equipment and operator experience.

Impact of guidelines and team composition

- Success rates for FONA have slightly improved since the 2017 UK guidelines, which emphasize surgical techniques. However, pooled rates before and after 2017 remained consistent at 88%.
- Physician-led teams achieved the highest crude median success rate of 100%, whereas military teams had the lowest at 81.5%. This discrepancy underscores the importance of advanced training and expertise in performing FONA.

Pediatric considerations

- Pediatric FONA success rates showed a median of 100%, but pooled data revealed lower reliability at 74%. Limited data and higher rates of complications, particularly with needle techniques, necessitate caution and further research.

Recommendations for practice

Technique selection

1. Prioritize surgical techniques: Surgical FONA is the most reliable method, especially in high-stakes prehospital scenarios.
   - Recommended equipment includes a scalpel, bougie, and 6.0 mm tracheal tube as per UK guidelines.
2. Avoid needle techniques when possible: The lower success rates and increased risk of complications, such as subcutaneous emphysema and barotrauma, make needle approaches less favorable.

Training and preparation

- Advanced training: All prehospital providers, including paramedics and flight teams, should receive hands-on training in surgical FONA to improve confidence and proficiency.
- Simulation-based learning: Regularly simulate CICO scenarios to ensure readiness under pressure.

Pediatric management

- Due to limited evidence and higher rates of complications in pediatric FONA, there is no definitive guidance on the optimal approach. Providers should be familiar with both surgical and needle-based techniques to address diverse clinical presentations, though further research is needed to establish best practices.
- The Difficult Airway Society (DAS) recommends percutaneous cannula cricothyroidotomy for children aged 1-8 years, but further evidence is needed to validate this practice.

Broader implications

This review highlights the critical importance of surgical FONA in prehospital airway management. While success rates remain high overall, discrepancies in outcomes based on technique, team composition, and patient population emphasize the need for standardization and ongoing education.

Future directions include:

- Establishing an international database to collect standardized FONA data would facilitate more robust future studies by providing a larger, more consistent dataset for analyzing outcomes, identifying best practices, and improving training programs.
- Addressing gaps in pediatric FONA research to refine guidelines and optimize techniques for younger patients.
- Expanding access to advanced airway training programs, particularly for military and rural emergency teams.

Key takeaways

- ☑ Surgical FONA is the gold standard for prehospital airway access, with a pooled success rate of 92% and a median success rate of 100%.
- ☑ Needle techniques are less reliable, with a pooled success rate of only 52%, underscoring the need for surgical expertise.
- ☑ Physician-led teams consistently achieve higher success rates, highlighting the importance of advanced training and experience.
- ☑ Pediatric FONA remains an area requiring further study, with data suggesting lower reliability than adult procedures.
- ☑ Prehospital providers should prioritize surgical techniques, enhance training programs, and adopt simulation-based learning to improve outcomes in FONA scenarios.

Additional recommended reading:

1. Morton S, Avery P, Kua J, et al. Success rate of prehospital emergency front-of-neck access (FONA): A systematic review and meta-analysis. Br J Anaesth. 2023;130(5):636-644. PMID: 36858888; PMCID: PMC10170392.
2. Frerk C, Mitchell VS, McNarry AF, et al. Difficult Airway Society 2015 guidelines for management of unanticipated difficult intubation in adults. Br J Anaesth. 2015;115(6):827-848. PMID: 26556848; PMCID: PMC4650961.
3. Duggan LV, Lockhart SL, Cook TM, O'Sullivan EP, Dare T, Baker PA. The Airway App: exploring the role of smartphone technology to capture emergency front-of-neck airway experiences internationally. Anaesthesia. 2018;73(6):703-710. PMID: 29533465

Emergency treatment of anaphylaxis

32

Why this topic is important

Anaphylaxis is a life-threatening systemic hypersensitivity reaction that requires rapid recognition and treatment to prevent serious outcomes, including death. It is characterized by airway, breathing, and circulation (ABC) problems, often with skin or mucosal symptoms. While the overall prognosis of anaphylaxis is good with timely intervention, failure to recognize or treat the condition appropriately can lead to fatal consequences.

The updated 2021 guidelines from the Resuscitation Council UK (RCUK) introduce significant advancements in the management of anaphylaxis. They address common pitfalls, refine treatment algorithms, and recommend evidence-based strategies. Given the increasing incidence of anaphylaxis globally, this update equips healthcare professionals with critical knowledge to improve patient outcomes.

Objectives of this update

- Review the latest recommendations for recognizing and treating anaphylaxis.
- Emphasize the role of intramuscular (IM) adrenaline and correct patient positioning.
- Discuss the management of refractory anaphylaxis and biphasic reactions.
- Clarify the roles of adjunctive treatments, such as antihistamines and corticosteroids.

What is new

- Stronger emphasis on the immediate administration of IM adrenaline as the first-line treatment.
- Clearer recommendations against the routine use of corticosteroids in managing anaphylaxis.
- Introduction of a treatment algorithm for refractory anaphylaxis, emphasizing intravenous (IV) adrenaline infusion.
- Refined guidelines on observation duration and discharge planning, incorporating risk stratification.

Key findings

Recognizing anaphylaxis

Anaphylaxis is a clinical diagnosis defined by its sudden onset and rapid progression, typically involving:

- ABC problems (e.g., airway swelling, bronchospasm, hypotension).
- Skin and mucosal changes (e.g., urticaria, angioedema) in most, but not all, cases.
- Gastrointestinal symptoms (e.g., vomiting, abdominal pain) can sometimes mimic or accompany other symptoms.

Correct recognition is crucial, as delays or misdiagnoses can lead to inappropriate treatment. Skin changes alone do not constitute anaphylaxis and should not delay interventions for ABC compromise.

First-line treatment: adrenaline

- IM adrenaline: The cornerstone of anaphylaxis treatment, administered as soon as the condition is identified.
    - Administer into the mid-anterolateral thigh, with a dose of 0.5 mg for adults.
    - Repeat every 5 minutes as needed if ABC problems persist.
- Delayed administration risks: Observational studies link delays in adrenaline administration to increased severity, higher risk of biphasic reactions, and mortality.
- IV adrenaline: Reserved for refractory cases and should only be administered by specialists in settings equipped for advanced monitoring due to the risk of complications like arrhythmias or stroke.

Adjunctive treatments

- Antihistamines: Useful for treating skin symptoms (urticaria, angioedema) after ABC stabilization but should never delay adrenaline administration. Non-sedating antihistamines (e.g., cetirizine) are preferred.
- Corticosteroids: They are no longer recommended for routine use as the evidence does not support their role in reducing symptom duration or preventing biphasic reactions. However, they may still have a role in managing anaphylaxis with poorly controlled asthma or refractory symptoms.

Managing refractory anaphylaxis

Defined as persistent ABC problems despite two appropriate doses of IM adrenaline, refractory anaphylaxis requires urgent intervention:

- Low-dose IV adrenaline infusion: This is more effective than repeated IM or IV boluses, and it is provided by experienced clinicians in critical care settings.
- Fluid resuscitation: Administer IV fluids to counteract the plasma extravasation and hypovolemia common in severe anaphylaxis.
- Adjunctive measures: Consider bronchodilators for severe bronchospasm and nebulized adrenaline for critical upper airway obstruction.

Observation and discharge planning

The updated guidelines advocate a risk-stratified approach to determining observation duration and discharge readiness:

- Minimum observation: 2 hours from symptom resolution for low-risk cases with rapid response to adrenaline.
- Extended observation: 6-12 hours for patients requiring multiple adrenaline doses or with a history of biphasic reactions.
- Prolonged monitoring: 12 hours or more for patients with severe initial reactions, ongoing asthma, or uncertain access to emergency care after discharge.

All patients must receive clear discharge instructions, adrenaline auto-injectors with training, and a referral to an allergy specialist.

Biphasic reactions

- Approximately 5% of anaphylaxis cases experience a biphasic reaction, where symptoms recur hours after initial resolution. Key risk factors include severe initial reactions, delayed adrenaline administration, and the need for multiple adrenaline doses.
- While fatal biphasic reactions are rare, clinicians should educate patients on the signs and symptoms of recurrence and provide adequate follow-up care.

Challenges in practice

Despite robust guidelines, many patients with anaphylaxis are undertreated or mismanaged:

- Adrenaline is underutilized, often replaced by less effective treatments like antihistamines or corticosteroids.
- Misdiagnosis due to unfamiliarity with atypical presentations can delay life-saving interventions.
- Adverse outcomes are associated with postural changes, such as standing from a supine position, which can exacerbate cardiovascular collapse.

Recommendations for improved outcomes

Education and training

- Ensure all healthcare providers are proficient in recognizing and treating anaphylaxis.
- Conduct simulation-based training to reinforce guideline adherence, focusing on the correct administration of IM adrenaline.

Systems improvement

- Equip emergency settings with adrenaline auto-injectors, IV fluid resuscitation kits, and appropriate monitoring equipment.
- Standardize protocols for recognizing and managing refractory anaphylaxis across healthcare facilities.

Public awareness

- Educate patients and caregivers on the importance of early adrenaline use, proper auto-injector technique, and when to seek emergency care.

Key takeaways

☑ Anaphylaxis is a medical emergency requiring rapid administration of IM adrenaline as the first-line treatment.

☑ Adjunctive treatments, such as antihistamines, are secondary and should never delay adrenaline.

☑ Corticosteroids are no longer recommended for routine use and should be reserved for select cases.

☑ Managing refractory anaphylaxis requires advanced care with IV adrenaline infusions and fluid resuscitation.

☑ A risk-stratified approach to observation and discharge planning enhances patient safety and prevents complications.

Additional recommended reading:

1. Whyte AF, Soar J, Dodd A, Hughes A, Sargant N, Turner PJ. Emergency treatment of anaphylaxis: concise clinical guidance. Clin Med (Lond). 2022;22(4):332-339. PMID: 35882481; PMCID: PMC9345203.

2. Turner PJ, Campbell DE. Epidemiology of severe anaphylaxis. Curr Opin Allergy Clin Immunol. 2016;16(5):441-50. PMID: 27490124; PMCID: PMC5325322.

3. Dodd A, Hughes A, Sargant N et al. Evidence update for the treatment of anaphylaxis. Resuscitation. 2021;163:86-96. PMID: 33895231; PMCID: PMC8139870.

Specialized airway management techniques

Airway management in patients with unstable cervical spines

33

Why this topic is important

Airway management in patients with an unstable cervical spine (C-spine) presents a unique and high-risk challenge in anesthesia. These patients are often at heightened risk of secondary spinal cord injury (SCI) due to cervical instability, which complicates even routine maneuvers like intubation and ventilation. Trauma accounts for a significant portion of these cases, with C-spine injuries occurring in approximately 3.5% of trauma patients, of whom 40% present with instability.

Despite longstanding recommendations to minimize C-spine movement during airway management, controversies persist about the best techniques and devices to achieve this goal. Recent advances in video laryngoscopy (VL), manual in-line stabilization (MILS), and innovations in immobilization strategies offer new opportunities to refine practices. A review by d'Arville et al. 2022 evaluates current evidence and emerging trends in managing airways in patients with unstable cervical spines, providing actionable insights for anesthesiologists facing these complex cases.

Objectives of this update

- To review the risks and challenges of airway management in unstable C-spines.
- To assess the relative effectiveness of different intubation devices and techniques.
- To examine controversies surrounding spinal immobilization and its role in airway management.

Key findings

Risks associated with unstable cervical spines

Airway management in unstable C-spines is fraught with challenges, including:

1. Cervical spine movement:
    - Intubation maneuvers such as jaw thrust or laryngoscopy risk exacerbating spinal instability.
    - Studies suggest even minor movements during intubation may contribute to SCI, though precise thresholds remain unclear.
2. Compromised outcomes:
    - Perioperative claims data indicate that airway management contributes to 11% of spinal cord injuries during surgery, rising to 22% in patients with pre-existing spinal instability.
3. Balancing priorities:
    - Clinicians must minimize spinal movement while addressing other risks, such as hypoxia, aspiration, and hemodynamic instability.

Innovations in intubation techniques

The emergence of new devices has significantly shaped the landscape of airway management for unstable cervical spines.

1. Video laryngoscopy (VL):
    - VL offers superior glottic visualization with reduced neck movement compared to direct laryngoscopy (DL).
    - Devices such as the C-MAC and GlideScope demonstrate higher first-pass intubation success rates in immobilized patients.
    - However, VL's benefits diminish when used alongside MILS, as reduced occipital-cervical movement does not always translate to improved outcomes.
2. Fiberoptic intubation (FOI):
    - Long regarded as the gold standard for minimizing cervical movement, FOI remains the preferred technique in awake intubations for unstable spines.
    - Studies comparing FOI with VL show comparable success rates but suggest FOI achieves lower cervical spine displacement.
3. Novel approaches:
    - Devices like the Airtraq and King Vision VL have shown promise in specific settings, though further research is needed to validate their clinical advantages.

Spinal immobilization: Reassessing rigid collars and MILS

1. Rigid cervical collars:
    - While traditionally used for spinal immobilization, rigid collars introduce risks such as increased intracranial pressure, pressure ulcers, and aspiration.
    - Recent guidelines, including from the Eastern Association for the Surgery of Trauma (EAST), recommend against routine collar use, particularly in penetrating trauma.
2. Manual in-line stabilization (MILS):
    - MILS remains widely taught and used to stabilize the cervical spine during intubation. However, evidence supporting its efficacy is weak.
    - MILS can complicate laryngoscopy by worsening glottic views and prolonging intubation times, potentially increasing other perioperative risks.
3. Emerging alternatives:
    - Soft foam collars and vacuum mattresses are gaining traction as less intrusive options for spinal immobilization. Early studies suggest these alternatives do not compromise spinal stability while reducing complications.

Recommendations for clinical practice

Based on current evidence, the following strategies can optimize airway management in patients with unstable cervical spines:

1. Preoperative planning:
    - Perform high-resolution imaging to assess the extent of instability.
    - For preemptive planning, engage a multidisciplinary team, including trauma and spinal surgeons.
2. Device selection:
    - Prefer VL or FOI based on the clinical scenario and operator expertise.
    - Use VL for improved visualization in unconscious patients and FOI for awake intubations requiring precise neck movement control.
3. Immobilization strategies:
    - Consider alternatives to rigid collars, such as MILS or soft cervical collars, to balance stability with practicality.
    - Avoid over-reliance on immobilization techniques that may hinder airway access or prolong procedures.
4. Training and simulation:
    - Regularly train teams on intubation techniques and immobilization strategies for unstable spines.
    - Incorporate simulation-based learning to improve proficiency in using devices like VL and FOI.
5. Minimizing cervical movement:
    - Aim for acceptable rather than perfect laryngoscopic views to reduce the need for repeated attempts.
    - Avoid excessive external maneuvers, such as jaw thrusts, that can exacerbate spinal instability.

Limitations and future directions

Despite advancements in device technology and technique, several gaps remain:

1. Weak evidence base:
    - Most studies rely on surrogate outcomes like cervical displacement rather than direct measures of SCI.
    - Larger, randomized trials are needed to assess patient-centered outcomes, such as neurological function and long-term recovery.
2. Applicability to real-world settings:
    - Many studies use cadaveric models or controlled environments, which may not reflect the complexities of acute trauma care.
3. Developing new endpoints:
    - Future research should focus on reliable metrics for assessing the impact of airway interventions on spinal cord injury.

Key takeaways

☑ Video laryngoscopy and fiberoptic intubation are effective options for managing airways in patients with unstable cervical spines, each with unique advantages.

☑ Rigid cervical collars are increasingly replaced by less invasive alternatives, such as soft collars and vacuum mattresses.

☑ Manual in-line stabilization remains a controversial practice. Its benefits are offset by challenges in maintaining glottic views and efficient intubation.

☑ Multidisciplinary planning, operator expertise, and judicious use of immobilization are essential to achieving optimal outcomes.

Additional recommended reading:

1. d'Arville A, Walker M, Lacey J, et al. Airway management in the adult patient with an unstable cervical spine. *Curr Opin Anesthesiol.* 2021;34:597-602. PMID: 34325462
2. Singleton BN, Morris FK, Yet B, et al. Effectiveness of intubation devices in patients with cervical spine immobilisation: A systematic review and network meta-analysis. *Br J Anaesth.* 2021;126:1055-1066. PMID: 33610262.
3. Wiles MD. Manual in-line stabilisation during tracheal intubation: Effective protection or harmful dogma? *Anaesthesia.* 2021;76:850-853. PMID: 33939842.

Airway management in patients with obstructive sleep apnea

34

Why this topic is important

Obstructive sleep apnea (OSA) is the most prevalent sleep-related breathing disorder, characterized by repeated upper airway collapse during sleep. Patients with OSA often present unique challenges during surgical airway management due to anatomical and physiological features that predispose them to a difficult airway. These include increased soft tissue surrounding the airway, reduced lung volumes, and heightened susceptibility to rapid oxygen desaturation.

The perioperative period poses additional risks, including airway obstruction, respiratory depression, and cardiovascular instability. If these challenges are not anticipated and managed proactively, they can lead to life-threatening complications such as hypoxemia, aspiration, or a cannot-intubate-cannot-oxygenate (CICO) scenario. Furthermore, the increasing prevalence of OSA, driven by rising obesity rates, makes it imperative for anesthesiologists to refine their approach to airway management in this population.

OSA is also frequently undiagnosed before surgery, with many patients needing to be made aware of their condition. This complicates perioperative planning and necessitates robust screening tools and standardized protocols to minimize risks. A multidisciplinary approach involving preoperative optimization, intraoperative vigilance, and meticulous postoperative care is essential to mitigate complications and ensure patient safety. This update synthesizes evidence-based strategies for managing the airway in OSA patients, informed by Seet et al. (2021).

Objectives of this update

- Examine the association between OSA and difficult airway management.
- Outline evidence-based techniques for optimizing airway management in OSA patients.
- Highlight perioperative precautions to minimize complications.

What is new

- Patients with OSA have a 3- to 4-fold higher risk of difficult intubation and mask ventilation.
- The STOP-Bang questionnaire is reliable for predicting difficult airways in OSA patients.
- Updated guidelines emphasize awake intubation, head-elevated positioning, and multimodal analgesia for safe perioperative care.

Key findings

Association between OSA and difficult airway

- Higher risk of airway challenges:
  - OSA increases the likelihood of difficult intubation, difficult mask ventilation, and combined airway difficulties.
  - These challenges are key contributors to reduced pharyngeal space and increased soft tissue volume.
- Severity correlation: The risk of airway complications rises with higher apnea-hypopnea index (AHI) scores, with severe OSA patients showing the highest incidence of difficult intubation.
- Combined effects: The interplay between anatomical factors (e.g., large tongue, increased neck circumference) and physiological issues (e.g., rapid desaturation) makes managing OSA patients particularly complex.

Preoperative assessment

STOP-Bang questionnaire:

The STOP-Bang questionnaire is an effective and widely used tool for identifying OSA and predicting airway difficulties. It assesses eight key factors:

1. **S**noring: Loud snoring?
2. **T**iredness: Feeling tired, fatigued, or sleepy during the day?
3. **O**bserved apnea: Has anyone observed you stop breathing during sleep?
4. **P**ressure: History of high blood pressure?
5. **B**MI: Body mass index > 35 kg/m^2?
6. **A**ge: Age > 50 years?
7. **N**eck circumference: Neck circumference > 40 cm?
8. **G**ender: Male?

A score ≥ 3 indicates a moderate-to-high risk for OSA and potential airway difficulties, warranting additional precautions, such as advanced airway management planning and perioperative monitoring.

Ultrasound assessment:

Recent evidence suggests that point-of-care ultrasound can assess tongue base thickness and retroglossal airway diameter, aiding in predicting airway difficulties in OSA patients.

Perioperative strategies

Preoxygenation and oxygenation techniques

- Preoxygenation: Extending the safe apnea period is critical in OSA patients. Proper preoxygenation increases oxygen reserves and delays desaturation during airway management. Aim for an end-tidal oxygen fraction of 0.87-0.90.
- Apneic oxygenation: Using high-flow nasal oxygen during intubation reduces the risk of desaturation. This approach is particularly effective in obese OSA patients and during prolonged airway manipulation.

Awake intubation

Preferred in patients with known or suspected difficult airways.

- Ensure airway topicalization with lidocaine within the safe dose range. For central airway procedures, review the maximum dose recommendations; some sources suggest ≤ 8.3 mg/kg.
- Use flexible bronchoscopy, video-laryngoscopy, or a combination of both for safe and controlled intubation. Minimal sedation and supplemental high-flow oxygen are critical for maintaining oxygenation.

Asleep intubation

- Preparation: Adequate preoxygenation, skilled assistance, and a difficult airway cart are prerequisites for successful asleep intubation.
- Positioning: Elevate the head to align the external auditory meatus with the sternal notch. This improves the laryngoscopic view and increases functional residual capacity.

- Videolaryngoscopy: This technique enhances glottic visualization and increases first-attempt success rates. It is particularly useful for managing difficult airways in OSA patients.

Postoperative considerations

Extubation strategies

- Anticipate challenges: Difficult extubation may occur due to residual airway edema, altered anatomy, or incomplete neuromuscular blockade reversal.
- Awake extubation: Extubate only when the patient is fully awake and cooperative. A semi-upright position minimizes airway collapse risks.
- Adjuncts: Airway exchange catheters and remifentanil infusions may provide additional safety during extubation.

Monitoring and oxygen therapy

- High-risk patients: Severe OSA patients, those undergoing upper airway surgeries, and those requiring high-dose opioids postoperatively should be closely monitored in high-acuity areas.
- Early CPAP therapy: To prevent postoperative airway obstruction, resume positive airway pressure therapy (e.g., CPAP or BiPAP) at the patient's prescribed settings as soon as feasible.

Analgesia and sedation

- Dexmedetomidine: A sedative with minimal or no respiratory depressant effects, making it a preferred choice in OSA patients. Avoid describing it as "short-acting."
- Multimodal analgesia reduces opioid use and associated respiratory risks.

Broader implications

Managing OSA patients requires a collaborative approach involving anesthesiologists, surgeons, and respiratory specialists. Integrating advanced screening tools, optimized perioperative care, and vigilant postoperative monitoring can significantly improve outcomes. Adopting personalized airway management strategies based on OSA severity and airway features will further enhance safety and effectiveness.

Key takeaways

☑ OSA significantly increases the risk of difficult intubation and mask ventilation.

☑ Comprehensive preoperative assessment improves airway risk prediction, including STOP-Bang scoring and ultrasound.

☑ Awake intubation is preferred in high-risk OSA patients with anticipated difficult airways.

☑ Postoperative monitoring and the early resumption of CPAP therapy are critical for preventing complications.

☑ Multimodal analgesia and careful sedation strategies minimize respiratory depression in OSA patients.

Additional recommended reading:

1. Seet E, Nagappa M, Wong DT. Airway Management in Surgical Patients With Obstructive Sleep Apnea. *Anesth Analg.* 2021;132(5):1321-1327. PMID: 33857974.

2. Memtsoudis SG, Cozowicz C, Nagappa M, et al. Society of Anesthesia and Sleep Medicine Guideline on Intraoperative Management of Adult Patients With Obstructive Sleep Apnea. Anesth Analg. 2018;127(4):967-987. PMID: 29944522; PMCID: PMC6135479.

3. Ahmad I, El-Boghdadly K, Bhagrath R, et al. Difficult Airway Society Guidelines for Awake Tracheal Intubation. *Anaesthesia.* 2020;75:509-528. PMID: 31729018; PMCID: PMC7078877.

Intraoperative airway management for patients with tracheostomy

35

Why this topic is important

Managing adult patients with tracheostomy during anesthesia presents unique challenges, including airway obstruction, accidental dislodgement, and stoma-related complications. Tracheostomies are often performed in patients with critical illnesses, upper airway obstructions, or as part of major head and neck surgeries. Intraoperative care for these patients requires tailored airway management strategies, as failure to secure the airway can lead to catastrophic consequences such as hypoxia, pneumothorax, or cardiac arrest.

A narrative review by Rosero et al. 2021 underscores the importance of understanding tracheostomy devices, pre-procedural assessments, and multidisciplinary collaboration to improve patient outcomes during surgery. Effective planning and execution can mitigate risks and ensure optimal care in this high-risk population.

Objectives of this update

- Outline key considerations for managing adult patients with tracheostomy under anesthesia.
- Discuss strategies for addressing tracheostomy-related emergencies, such as tube dislodgement or obstruction.
- Provide actionable recommendations for selecting and using tracheostomy devices intraoperatively.

What is new

- A structured preoperative checklist ensures a thorough assessment of tracheostomy-related factors, including stoma maturity, device type, and patient positioning.
- Detailed guidelines for managing patients with specific devices, such as T-tubes or uncuffed tracheostomy tubes, are highlighted.
- An algorithm for managing tracheostomy tube dislodgement during anesthesia offers a practical tool for emergency response.

Key findings

Preoperative considerations

1. Comprehensive preoperative checklist:
    - Evaluate the indication for the tracheostomy, as it determines whether oral intubation is possible in emergencies.
    - Assess the timing of the tracheostomy; recent procedures (< 7 days) may have immature stomas, increasing the risk of complications during tube exchange.
    - Consider patient-specific factors, such as coagulation status, obesity, and respiratory conditions, which may impact airway management.
2. Stoma and device assessment:
    - Mature stomas are less prone to complications during tube exchange and are preferred for prolonged anesthesia cases.
    - The type of tracheostomy device-cuffed versus uncuffed, fenestrated versus non-fenestrated-determines the feasibility of positive pressure ventilation and potential airway obstructions.
3. Collaboration and preparation:
    - Early involvement of an otolaryngologist is critical, especially for patients with complex anatomy or T-tubes.
    - Ensure availability of backup airway equipment, including flexible bronchoscopes, tracheal tube exchangers, and pediatric facemasks for stoma ventilation.

Intraoperative management

1. Using the existing tracheostomy tube:
    - If cuffed tracheostomy tubes are securely positioned and function properly, they may suffice for short procedures in the supine position.
    - Connect dual-cannula tubes to the anesthesia circuit using the inner cannula's 15-mm adapter to minimize airway resistance.
2. Exchanging tracheostomy tubes for endotracheal tubes:
    - The exchange may be necessary for prone positioning, lengthy surgeries, or using devices like laser-resistant tracheal tubes.
    - Perform the exchange under topical anesthesia and minimal sedation to ensure spontaneous respiration until proper placement is confirmed.
3. Special device considerations:
    - T-tubes: Positive pressure ventilation through T-tubes can be challenging due to leaks and device anatomy. Options include using a cuffed tracheal tube or jet ventilation with a rigid bronchoscope in the external limb.
    - Stomal maintenance devices: Replace stents or buttons with cuffed tracheostomy or tracheal tubes to ensure secure ventilation during anesthesia.

Tracheostomy emergencies

1. Tube obstruction or dislodgement:
    - If airway pressures rise or oxygenation worsens suspect obstruction. Confirm patency by passing a suction catheter through the tube.
    - For recent tracheostomies, avoid forceful reinsertion to prevent creating a false passage. Flexible bronchoscopy can guide proper placement.
2. Algorithm for dislodgement management:
    - Prioritize oxygenation via mask or stoma ventilation while preparing for definitive airway access.
    - Mature stomas allow for the reinsertion of a smaller tracheal tube, while oral intubation is preferable for immature stomas.

Recommendations for practice

Preoperative strategies

- Use a checklist: Standardize preoperative evaluations with a checklist that includes stoma maturity, tracheostomy type, patient anatomy, and procedural positioning.
- Anticipate complications: Identify potential challenges, such as bleeding risks or limited ventilation options, and ensure appropriate equipment is available.

Intraoperative techniques

- Optimize device selection: Tailor tracheostomy or tracheal tube selection to the patient's anatomy and procedural needs, considering reinforced or laser-resistant tubes for specialized cases.
- Ensure secure ventilation: To prevent ventilation interruptions, regularly check tube connections, cuff pressures, and stoma patency during the procedure.

Multidisciplinary collaboration

- Engage specialists: Collaborate with oto-laryngologists, particularly for patients with complex airway conditions or rare devices like T-tubes.
- Train staff: Enhance team readiness with simulation training on tracheostomy management and emergency scenarios.

Broader implications

The management of tracheostomy patients during anesthesia requires a meticulous, multidisciplinary approach to prevent complications. This review highlights the importance of standardized protocols, advanced planning, and familiarity with various tracheostomy devices. As the prevalence of tracheostomy patients increases due to prolonged critical care, these strategies will remain essential for ensuring safe and effective perioperative care.

Future directions include:

- Expanding research on best practices for managing rare devices like T-tubes.
- Developing predictive tools to assess risks associated with specific tracheostomy conditions.
- Incorporating advanced airway simulation programs into routine anesthesia training.

Key takeaways

☑ Thorough preoperative assessments, including a checklist, are crucial for tracheostomy management under anesthesia.

☑ Tailored airway strategies should consider the type of tracheostomy device, stoma maturity, and patient-specific factors like positioning or coagulation status.

☑ Managing emergencies such as tube obstruction or dislodgement requires a structured algorithm prioritizing oxygenation and careful airway re-establishment.

☑ Multidisciplinary collaboration and continuous education are key to improving outcomes for this high-risk population.

Additional recommended reading:

1. Rosero EB, Corbett J, Mau T, Joshi GP. Intraoperative airway management considerations for adult patients presenting with tracheostomy: a narrative review. *Anesth Analg*. 2021;132(4):1003-1011. PMID: 33369928.

2. McGrath BA, Wallace S, Lynch J, et al. Improving tracheostomy care in the UK: Results of a guided quality improvement programme. *Br J Anaesth*. 2020;125:e119-e129. PMID: 32493580.

3. Oliveira VM, Weschenfelder ME, Deponti G, et al. Good practices for prone positioning at the bedside: Construction of a care protocol. Rev Assoc Med Bras (1992). 2016;62(3):287-293. PMID: 27310555.

Supraglottic airway devices in cesarean sections under general anesthesia

36

Why this topic is important

Airway management in obstetric patients undergoing general anesthesia presents unique challenges. Physiological changes during pregnancy, such as reduced functional residual capacity and increased oxygen demand, create a limited tolerance for apnea. Additionally, hormonal and mechanical changes increase the risk of pulmonary aspiration. Tracheal intubation is traditionally considered the gold standard for securing the airway in such cases, but it comes with risks of failed intubation and hemodynamic instability.

The emergence of second-generation supraglottic airway (SGA) devices offers an alternative for airway management in specific patient populations. These devices are designed to provide effective ventilation and protect against aspiration. Their use in cesarean sections has garnered interest due to their ease of insertion, faster time to effective ventilation, and favorable hemodynamic profile. Sanganee et al. (2024) conducted a comprehensive review to evaluate the evidence supporting SGA use in obstetric patients and propose a framework for its appropriate application.

Objectives of this update

- Assess the evidence supporting the use of SGAs in cesarean sections under general anaesthesia.
- Identify patient populations for whom SGAs may be appropriate.
- To guide integrating SGAs into clinical practice safely and effectively.

What is new

- Second-generation SGAs, such as the ProSeal, Supreme, and i-gel, demonstrated high first-attempt success rates of up to 99%.
- Time to effective ventilation was significantly faster with SGAs than with tracheal intubation, particularly in low-risk patients.
- The risk of pulmonary aspiration remains a concern, though reported adverse events are rare.

Key findings

Safety and efficacy of SGAs

- High insertion success: In observational and randomized controlled trials, second-generation SGAs showed a first-attempt insertion success rate ranging from 98% to 99%. When failures occurred, conversion to tracheal intubation was rare.
- Time to ventilation: SGAs reduced the time to effective ventilation by approximately 22 seconds compared to intubation, which could be crucial in emergencies.
- Pulmonary aspiration risk: Despite physiological safeguards in SGA design, there is limited evidence to confirm reduced aspiration risk. In over 7000 cases reviewed, only one instance of gastric regurgitation was documented, with no reported cases of aspiration.

Comparative outcomes with tracheal intubation

- Tracheal intubation remains the gold standard due to its superior aspiration protection. However, it is associated with greater hemodynamic changes during insertion and removal.
- SGAs demonstrated smoother hemodynamic profiles, with fewer incidents of hypertension or tachycardia.

Patient selection criteria

- Favorable candidates: SGAs are most appropriate for fasted, non-obese patients with no significant comorbidities or difficult airway predictors.
- Contraindications: Patients with elevated aspiration risk (e.g., unfasted, GERD, high BMI) or predicted difficult intubation may not be suitable candidates for SGA use.

Recommendations for clinical practice

Integrating SGAs into obstetric anaesthesia

1. Patient selection: Limit SGA use to low-risk parturients undergoing elective or emergency cesarean sections. Ensure thorough airway assessments and aspiration risk evaluations preoperatively.
2. Device choice: Second-generation SGAs are preferred due to their higher oropharyngeal leak pressures and ability to accommodate gastric tubes for aspiration of stomach contents.
3. Insertion technique: Use rapid sequence induction with neuromuscular blockade to facilitate SGA placement. Preoxygenate patients and consider high-flow nasal oxygen to extend apnoea time during insertion.

Training and resource allocation

- Ensure that all clinicians involved in obstetric airway management are proficient in SGA insertion and troubleshooting.
- Equip delivery units with second-generation SGAs and adjunctive devices like video laryngoscopes for backup.

Broader implications

The findings from this review underscore the potential of SGAs to serve as an alternative to tracheal intubation in selected obstetric patients. Their use could reduce procedural complexity, improve hemodynamic stability, and expedite ventilation. However, tracheal intubation should remain the preferred option for high-risk scenarios until further evidence supports broader SGA adoption.

Future research should focus on:

- Large-scale trials to compare aspiration risk between SGAs and intubation.
- Evaluating the use of SGAs in diverse patient populations, including those with obesity or gestational diabetes.
- Incorporating gastric ultrasound into preoperative assessments to better stratify aspiration risk.

Key takeaways

☑ Second-generation SGAs provide a viable alternative to tracheal intubation in carefully selected parturients undergoing cesarean sections.

☑ They offer high success rates, faster ventilation times, and improved hemodynamic profiles.

☑ Their use should be restricted to low-risk patients, with tracheal intubation reserved for higher-risk scenarios.

☑ Training and standardized protocols are essential to ensure the safe integration of SGAs into obstetric anesthesia practices.

Additional recommended reading:

1. Sanganee U, Jansen K, Lucas N, Van de Velde M. The role of supraglottic airway devices for caesarean section under general anaesthesia: A scoping literature review. Eur J Anaesthesiol. 2024;41:668—676. PMID: 38898775.
2. White LD, Thang C, Hodsdon A, et al. Comparison of supraglottic airway devices with endotracheal intubation in low-risk patients for caesarean delivery. Anesth Analg. 2020;131:1092-1101. PMID: 32925330.
3. McDonnell NJ, Paech MJ, Clavisi OM, Scott KL. Difficult and failed intubation in obstetric anaesthesia: An observational study. Int J Obstet Anesth. 2008;17:292-297. PMID: 18617389.

Video double-lumen tubes in thoracic surgery

37

Why this topic is important

Double-lumen tubes (DLTs) are essential for achieving one-lung ventilation during thoracic surgery, but their use is associated with complications like airway injuries, postoperative sore throat, and hoarseness. Video double-lumen tubes (VDLTs), which include an embedded camera for continuous visualization, have emerged as a potential alternative to traditional DLTs. VDLTs aim to enhance procedural safety and reduce complications by improving intubation accuracy. Additionally, VDLTs offer continuous visualization of the carina and trachea, providing intraoperative advantages during bronchial surgeries and other complex procedures.

The 2024 study by Shui et al. evaluates the clinical impact of VDLTs compared to DLTs in thoracic surgery. This update summarizes the study's findings and addresses the benefits, limitations, and implications of VDLTs in clinical practice.

Objectives of this update

- Examine the effectiveness and safety of VDLTs versus traditional DLTs.
- Highlight key findings related to intubation success, airway injuries, and postoperative complications.
- Explore intraoperative and postoperative benefits and challenges associated with VDLTs.
- Provide recommendations for integrating VDLTs into clinical practice.

What is new

- VDLTs significantly improve intubation success rates and reduce intubation time compared to DLTs.
- VDLTs provide real-time imaging of the carina and trachea, aiding bronchial surgeries and facilitating lung isolation with video single-lumen tubes (SLTs) or bronchial blockers.
- VDLTs are associated with a higher incidence of transient sore throat and hoarseness compared to DLTs.

Key findings

Intubation success and efficiency

- First-attempt success rates: VDLTs achieved significantly higher success rates (91.3%) than DLTs (14.4%), reducing the need for repeated attempts.
- Intubation time: VDLTs shortened the time required for successful intubation (median 96 seconds) compared to DLTs (median 138 seconds), attributed to the embedded camera allowing real-time visualization.

Airway injuries and complications

- Tracheal injuries: Moderate-to-severe injuries occurred in 48.9% of patients with VDLTs and 35.6% with DLTs, though the difference was not statistically significant.
- Vocal cord injuries: Similar rates were reported between groups (VDLTs: 37%, DLTs: 34.4%), indicating no additional risk from VDLTs.
- Postoperative sore throat and hoarseness:
    - Sore throat: More common with VDLTs at 24 hours post-surgery (38%) compared to DLTs (23.3%).
    - Hoarseness: At 24 hours, VDLTs had higher rates (54.3%) than DLTs (36.6%).
    - Symptoms largely resolved by 48 hours, suggesting short-term effects.

Intraoperative benefits

- Continuous visualization: VDLTs enable real-time monitoring of the carina and trachea, facilitating optimal positioning during lung isolation procedures and allowing rapid correction of bronchial misplacement.
- Bronchial surgery: The embedded camera improves procedural control during bronchial resections or reconstructions.
- Lung isolation: VDLTs simplify the placement of video-guided SLTs and bronchial blockers for selective lung ventilation.

Safety outcomes

- Hypoxemia: VDLTs reduced hypoxemia during intubation (3.3% incidence) compared to DLTs (21.1%), likely due to faster and more accurate placement.
- Bronchial misplacement: Misplacement rates were lower with VDLTs (3.3%) than DLTs (12.2%), reducing the need for repositioning and associated risks.

Challenges and limitations

- Postoperative discomfort: The larger outer diameter and rigidity of VDLTs contribute to higher rates of sore throat and hoarseness, though symptoms are self-limiting.
- Airway injuries: While not statistically significant, the higher incidence of moderate-to-severe tracheal injuries with VDLTs underscores the need for cautious handling.
- Loss of image quality: Secretions can obscure the camera lens, particularly during prolonged surgeries, limiting visualization and requiring additional interventions to maintain clarity.

Recommendations for practice

Patient selection

- Use VDLTs for cases requiring high precision, such as surgeries involving complex airway anatomy or when rapid intubation is critical.

Technique optimization

- Ensure proper tube size selection based on tracheal dimensions to minimize airway trauma.
- Combine VDLTs with fiberoptic bronchoscopy as needed to confirm placement and maintain visualization during surgeries.

Intraoperative strategies

- Use suction to clear secretions from the camera lens to maintain image quality.
- Leverage the continuous visualization capability to monitor airway structures and ensure accurate lung isolation.

Managing postoperative complications

- Monitor patients for sore throat and hoarseness and provide symptomatic relief with analgesics or anti-inflammatory agents.
- Educate patients about the transient nature of these symptoms to alleviate concerns.

Training and standardization

- Train anesthesiologists in using VDLTs properly, emphasizing careful insertion techniques to reduce the risk of injuries.
- Standardize protocols for VDLT handling, including preoperative assessments to guide tube selection and postoperative care.

Broader implications for airway management

Integrating VDLTs into clinical practice reflects a broader trend toward leveraging visualization technology to improve procedural outcomes. While VDLTs offer clear advantages in precision and efficiency, their adoption should be accompanied by strategies to address associated complications.

Future research should focus on refining VDLT design to minimize discomfort, investigating long-term outcomes of airway injuries, and exploring cost-effectiveness in different healthcare settings. These efforts will ensure that VDLTs are used optimally to enhance patient safety and satisfaction.

Key takeaways

- ☑ VDLTs improve first-attempt success rates and reduce intubation time, enhancing procedural efficiency.
- ☑ Continuous visualization provides intraoperative benefits for complex thoracic procedures, including bronchial surgeries and lung isolation.
- ☑ Postoperative sore throat and hoarseness are more common with VDLTs but resolve within 48 hours.
- ☑ Image degradation due to secretions remains a challenge, requiring intraoperative management strategies.
- ☑ VDLTs are particularly beneficial in complex or emergency thoracic surgeries requiring high precision and speed.

Additional recommended reading:

1. Shui W, Hu W, Ma W, et al. The effects of video double-lumen tubes on intubation complications in patients undergoing thoracic surgery. *Eur J Anaesthesiol*. 2024;41:305-313. PMID: 38298060; PMCID: PMC10906194.
2. Heir JS, Guo SL, et al. Intubation with video double-lumen tubes: A randomized controlled study. *J Cardiothorac Vasc Anesth*. 2018;32:267-274. PMID: 29074128.
3. Levy-Faber D, Malyanker Y, et al. Comparing VivaSight double-lumen tubes and conventional double-lumen tubes in thoracic surgery. *Anaesthesia*. 2015;70:1259-1263. PMID: 26192743.

Laryngeal keel placement for airway management

38

Why this topic is important

Laryngeal keels are crucial surgical devices used to treat glottic webs and prevent complications such as scarring and airway stenosis. These keels are typically placed following glottic web excision to maintain separation between the raw mucosal edges of the anterior commissure. While effective in promoting healing and improving voice outcomes, their presence introduces unique challenges for anesthetic management, especially during placement, removal, or emergency intubation.

Understanding the implications of laryngeal keels is critical for anesthesiologists to ensure patient safety and procedural success. Improper management can result in complications like keel displacement, granulation tissue formation, or airway compromise, which could lead to severe outcomes. Kirti et al. (2024) outline key considerations for managing airways in patients with laryngeal keels, emphasizing the need for specialized strategies and heightened vigilance during airway manipulation.

Objectives of this update

- Highlight the purpose and surgical applications of laryngeal keels in glottic web management.
- Review challenges and complications associated with airway management in patients with laryngeal keels.
- Provide evidence-based recommendations to optimize perioperative and emergency airway strategies for such patients.

What is new

- Gore-Tex is increasingly used as a laryngeal keel material due to its biocompatibility and efficacy in promoting near-perfect healing and improved voice outcomes.
- Recent cases emphasize the risks of keel displacement and iatrogenic aspiration, underscoring the importance of meticulous airway management during intubation or manipulation.
- Updated recommendations advocate for smaller endotracheal tubes (ETTs), intravenous steroids, and alternative airway strategies to prevent complications.

Key findings

Purpose and placement of laryngeal keels

- Primary goal: Laryngeal keels prevent glottic web recurrence by separating anterior commissures.
- Materials and methods: Keels are fashioned from biocompatible materials such as Gore-Tex, Teflon, or silicone and are secured via sutures either endoscopically or through open approaches.
- Surgical technique:
  - Endoscopic methods involve transoral scar lysis and keel placement secured to the anterior neck.
  - Open approaches use a transcervical laryngofissure and stiffer keels directly sutured to the thyroid cartilage.

Anesthetic challenges and strategies

1. Perioperative considerations
   - Glottic repairs often result in significant laryngeal edema, necessitating strategies to maintain airway patency and prevent obstruction.
   - Administering intravenous steroids preoperatively helps reduce inflammation and improve visualization during the procedure.
2. Airway management during keel presence
   - Smaller-than-expected ETTs should be employed to avoid disturbing the keel and to accommodate swelling.
   - Avoiding supraglottic airway devices is critical, as these may displace the keel or fail to provide a definitive airway.
   - If displacement occurs, rigid bronchoscopy may be required to retrieve the keel and manage complications.
3. Emergency scenarios
   - Keel dislodgement may lead to airway compromise, requiring rapid establishment of a definitive airway.
   - Though rare, keel aspiration can result in distal airway obstruction or granulation tissue formation, necessitating urgent removal via bronchoscopy.

Risks and complications

- Keel displacement and adhesion formation: Displacement risks improper healing, potentially causing scarring and airway stenosis.
- Iatrogenic aspiration: The aspiration of a displaced keel can obstruct distal airways, leading to respiratory distress.
- Inadequate healing: Failure to manage keels appropriately during airway manipulation may compromise surgical outcomes, including voice quality and airway patency.

Recommendations for practice

Perioperative management

1. Anesthetic induction: Prefer natural airway with spontaneous respiration to minimize keel disturbance.
2. ETT selection: Use smaller ETTs during intubation to avoid keel contact and confirm tube placement with careful visualization.
3. Medication: Administer intravenous steroids to reduce laryngeal edema preoperatively.

Emergency interventions

- Definitive airway: Establish a secure airway without relying on supraglottic devices, as these are contraindicated in keel displacement.
- Bronchoscopy: Maintain readiness for rigid bronchoscopy to address complications like keel aspiration or severe stenosis.

Postoperative care

- Monitor for signs of keel displacement or airway compromise during recovery and schedule timely follow-ups for keel removal (typically 3-5 weeks post-placement).

Broader implications

- The presence of laryngeal keels highlights the complexities of airway management in patients with surgically altered anatomy. Anesthesiologists play a pivotal role in ensuring the success of these interventions by tailoring strategies to the unique challenges posed by keels.

Future directions include:

- Standardizing protocols for airway management in patients with laryngeal keels to minimize variability in care.
- Researching alternative materials and designs to reduce the risks of complications further.
- Incorporating simulation training into anesthesiology education to improve proficiency in managing airways with laryngeal modifications.

Key takeaways

☑ Laryngeal keels prevent scarring and stenosis following glottic web excision but introduce significant airway management challenges.

☑ Smaller ETTs, avoidance of supraglottic devices, and preoperative steroid administration are key strategies for safe airway management.

☑ Displacement or aspiration of keels can lead to severe complications requiring rigid bronchoscopy and definitive airway establishment.

☑ Collaboration between anesthesiologists and otolaryngologists is critical to optimizing outcomes and managing potential complications effectively.

Additional recommended reading:

1. Kirti S, Fuhrmann M, Ok MS. Laryngeal keel and its implications during airway management. *Anesthesiology*. 2024;141:159-160. PMID: 38498666.
2. Nicollas R, Triglia JM. The anterior laryngeal webs. *Otolaryngol Clin North Am*. 2008;41:877-888. PMID: 18775339.
3. Sharouny H, Omar RB. Iatrogenic aspiration of custom-made keel: A case report. *Iran Red Crescent Med J*. 2014;16:e17066. PMID: 25763237; PMCID: PMC4341253.

Complex airway management in Mounier-Kuhn syndrome with tracheal diverticula

39

Why this topic is important

Airway management is a cornerstone of anesthetic practice, particularly in patients with challenging airway anatomy. Mounier-Kuhn syndrome, also known as tracheobronchomegaly, presents unique challenges due to marked tracheal and bronchial dilation caused by thinning or atrophy of the tracheal elastic fibers and smooth muscle. This rare condition can be complicated further by tracheal diverticula-outpouchings in the tracheal wall that act as reservoirs for secretions and exacerbate airway compromise.

Complications like excessive air leaks and ineffective ventilation can arise during mechanical ventilation due to tracheal dilation and the inability of standard endotracheal tubes (ETTs) to form an adequate seal. These risks highlight the importance of tailored strategies in airway management for such patients. A recent report by Chao et al. 2024 details a case of a 52-year-old man with Mounier-Kuhn syndrome undergoing laparoscopic colectomy, where innovative approaches were required to manage multiple tracheal diverticula and achieve successful ventilation.

Objectives of this update

- To explore airway management challenges in patients with Mounier-Kuhn syndrome complicated by tracheal diverticula.
- Describe practical solutions for overcoming issues such as air leaks and ventilation inefficiency.
- To highlight the importance of preoperative planning and intraoperative flexibility in managing complex airway cases.

Case summary

A 52-year-old male with a known history of Mounier-Kuhn syndrome was scheduled for laparoscopic colectomy. Preoperative computed tomography (CT) scans revealed tracheal dilation with a transverse tracheal diameter exceeding 30 mm and multiple tracheal diverticula. The right and left main bronchi measured 24 mm and 23 mm, respectively, meeting the diagnostic criteria for Mounier-Kuhn syndrome.

After induction of general anesthesia, a 7.5-mm ETT was inserted, but significant peritubal air leaks occurred during mechanical ventilation. The problem persisted despite replacing the tube with an 8.0-mm ETT and excessively inflating the cuff. Flexible bronchoscopy identified multiple tracheal diverticula, and repositioning the tube beyond the diverticula reduced the air leak to clinically acceptable levels. Ventilation was maintained successfully, and the patient recovered uneventfully.

Key challenges and solutions

Air leaks and ventilation challenges

1. Problem:
    - Excessive tracheal dilation in Mounier-Kuhn syndrome prevents standard ETT cuffs from forming an adequate seal, leading to air leaks and inadequate ventilation.
    - Tracheal diverticula further complicate sealing and increase the risk of aspiration and ineffective ventilation.
2. Solution:
    - Subglottic placement of a larger ETT: An 8.0-mm ETT was positioned beyond the tracheal diverticula to minimize air leaks.
    - Excessive cuff inflation: While not ideal, this approach was necessary to limit leakage to acceptable levels.

Secretions and airway hygiene

1. Problem:
    - Diverticula act as reservoirs for secretions, increasing the risk of aspiration and respiratory infections.
2. Solution:
    - Flexible bronchoscopy was used intraoperatively to suction secretions from the diverticula and optimize ventilation.

Preoperative planning

1. Problem:
    - Without careful preoperative imaging, airway abnormalities in Mounier-Kuhn syndrome can go unrecognized, leading to intraoperative complications.
2. Solution:
    - High-resolutio CT imaging was instrumental in diagnosing tracheal diverticula and planning airway management strategies.

Clinical implications

Tailored airway management

Patients with Mounier-Kuhn syndrome require individualized airway management plans. Key considerations include:

- Preoperative imaging: Routine CT scans should be considered for patients with known or suspected airway abnormalities.
- Flexible bronchoscopy: This tool is invaluable for assessing tracheal anatomy and identifying diverticula during intubation.
- Customizing ETT selection: Larger-diameter or cuff-modified ETTs can help address tracheal dilation.

Risks of excessive cuff inflation

While cuff inflation can minimize leaks, excessive pressure risks tracheal injury or ischemia, continuous monitoring of cuff pressures and using alternatives such as wet gauze to seal the throat may reduce these risks.

Multidisciplinary collaboration

Effective management requires coordination between anesthesiologists, surgeons, and pulmonologists to address the multifaceted challenges posed by Mounier-Kuhn syndrome.

Recommendations for practice

1. Preoperative evaluation:
    - Obtain high-resolution imaging to assess tracheal diameter and detect diverticula.
    - Involve a multidisciplinary team early in planning.
2. Intraoperative strategies:
    - Use flexible bronchoscopy to guide tube placement and manage secretions.
    - Position the ETT beyond the tracheal diverticula whenever feasible.
    - Be prepared to use larger or specially designed ETTs to address tracheal dilation.
3. Postoperative care:
    - Monitor closely for complications like tracheal injury, aspiration, or respiratory infections.
    - Consider follow-up with pulmonology for airway hygiene and long-term management.

Key takeaways

☑ Mounier-Kuhn syndrome complicates airway management due to tracheal dilation and diverticula, increasing the risk of air leaks and ventilation challenges.

☑ Preoperative imaging and intraoperative bronchoscopy are critical tools for optimizing airway strategies.

☑ Tailored approaches, such as larger ETTs and excessive cuff inflation, can mitigate air leaks but require careful monitoring to prevent complications.

☑ Multidisciplinary collaboration is essential to ensure safe and effective management.

Additional recommended reading:

1. Chao L, Zhang L, Yu J, Miao C. Complicated airway management because of multiple tracheal diverticula in a patient with Mounier-Kuhn syndrome. *Anesthesiology*. 2024;140(2):291-292. PMID: 38063471.
2. Mondoni M, Carlucci P, Parazzini EM, et al. Huge tracheal diverticulum in a patient with Mounier-Kuhn syndrome. *Eur J Case Rep Intern Med*. 2016;3:000419. PMID: 30755880; PMCID: PMC6346966.
3. Min JJ, Lee JM, Kim JH, et al. Anesthetic management of a patient with Mounier-Kuhn syndrome undergoing off-pump coronary artery bypass graft surgery: A case report. *Korean J Anesthesiol*. 2011;61:83-87. PMID: 21860757; PMCID: PMC3155143.

Education and technology in airway management

Teaching airway management using virtual reality

40

Why this topic is important

Airway management is a core skill for anesthesiologists and critical care providers, essential for ensuring safe ventilation and oxygenation in routine and emergency scenarios. Traditionally, airway management training has followed an apprenticeship model, where skills are acquired through observation, practice, and feedback during clinical exposure. However, this approach is increasingly constrained by reduced trainee work hours, fewer opportunities for high-risk case exposure, and an emphasis on patient safety.

Virtual reality (VR) simulation presents a transformative opportunity to overcome these limitations. By creating immersive and interactive learning environments, VR can replicate real-world conditions without exposing patients to risk. This update explores the potential of VR as a tool for airway management training, emphasizing its applications, benefits, and the need for standardized metrics to integrate it effectively into medical education.

Objectives of this update

- Summarize current applications of VR in airway management training.
- Highlight its advantages over traditional teaching methods and simulation modalities.
- Identify challenges and recommendations for integrating VR into structured training programs.

What is new

A scoping review of 15 studies on VR in airway management revealed that VR simulations significantly enhance skill acquisition and user satisfaction compared to didactic and traditional simulation methods. However, these studies highlight a lack of standardization in protocols, metrics, and integration into formal curricula. This gap underscores the need for guidelines from professional societies to maximize VR's educational potential.

Current applications of VR in airway management

Procedures simulated

The reviewed studies by Duffy et al. covered a range of airway techniques, including:

- **Flexible fibreoptic intubation (FOI):** The most commonly studied skill, involving intricate endoscopic navigation.
- **Direct and video laryngoscopy:** Techniques for tracheal intubation, focusing on glottic visualization and first-pass success.
- **Emergency cricothyrotomy:** A life-saving front-of-neck procedure in failed airway scenarios.

VR modalities

- **Immersive virtual reality (IVR):** Headset-based simulations providing high-fidelity experiences with visual, auditory, and sometimes haptic feedback.
- **Augmented reality (AR):** Overlaying virtual elements on the physical environment to assist with tasks like video laryngoscopy.
- **Mixed reality (MR):** Combining IVR and AR to create hybrid training scenarios.

Examples include:

- The ORSIM virtual bronchoscopy simulator for FOI.
- The GI-Bronch Mentor mannequin, integrating VR and physical task training.
- Augmented reality-assisted video laryngoscopy using smart glasses.

Comparison to traditional training

Many studies compared VR to didactic teaching, task trainers, and high-fidelity mannequin-based simulation. VR consistently demonstrated:

- Faster acquisition of procedural skills.
- Higher participant engagement and satisfaction.
- Comparable or superior performance outcomes, particularly for novices.

Advantages of VR in airway management training

1. **Asynchronous learning:** VR enables trainees to practice independently, reducing reliance on faculty availability and clinical case exposure.
2. **Reproducibility:** Unlike clinical settings, VR allows repetitive practice of the same scenarios under standardized conditions.
3. **Safe environment:** Learners can make mistakes without risk to patients, fostering confidence and skill refinement.
4. **Realistic simulation:** High-quality VR platforms replicate clinical conditions with audiovisual cues and haptic feedback.
5. **Objective assessment:** VR platforms can track performance metrics, such as time to task completion, accuracy, and economy of motion, providing objective feedback.

Challenges in integrating VR into training

1. **Lack of standardization:**
    - Current studies lack uniform metrics for evaluating VR's effectiveness.
    - Outcome definitions (e.g., successful intubation) and assessment tools vary widely, complicating comparisons across studies.
2. **Cost and accessibility:**
    - VR systems can be expensive, and smaller institutions may struggle with the initial investment.
    - Maintenance and updates of software and hardware add to the financial burden.
3. **Technological limitations:**

- Cyber motion sickness, reported in some studies, can affect user tolerance and experience.

- The fidelity of some VR simulations may still fall short of replicating complex clinical scenarios.

4. **Integration into curricula:**
   - VR is rarely part of formal training programs and is often used ad hoc without clear guidelines or pathways for educators.
   - Multispecialty involvement in airway management complicates creating unified curricula.

Recommendations for implementation

Standardization and guidelines

- Professional societies, such as the American Society of Anesthesiologists and the Difficult Airway Society, should develop consensus guidelines for VR-based airway training. These should include:
  - Standardized performance metrics.
  - Defined competencies for different training levels (e.g., novice, intermediate, expert).
  - Recommendations for blending VR with other training modalities.

Research and development

- Conduct multicenter trials to validate VR's impact on real-world clinical outcomes.
- Explore advanced features, such as adaptive learning algorithms, to customize training to individual needs.
- Incorporate emerging technologies like artificial intelligence to enhance assessment and feedback.

Integration into curricula

- Use VR as a supplement, not a replacement, for clinical exposure and high-fidelity simulation.
- Incorporate VR into structured airway management courses, such as Fundamentals of Airway Management.
- Regularly schedule VR training sessions to prevent skill decay and update trainees on new techniques.

Key takeaways

☑ VR simulation is an innovative and effective tool for airway management training, particularly for FOI and emergency procedures.

☑ It offers unique advantages, including asynchronous learning, safe practice environments, and objective performance feedback.

☑ Challenges, such as cost, accessibility, and lack of standardization, must be addressed to maximize its impact.

☑ Professional societies and educators should lead efforts to integrate VR into formal curricula and establish standardized metrics for its use.

Additional recommended reading:

1. Duffy CC, Bass GA, Yi W, et al. Teaching airway management using virtual reality: a scoping review. *Anesth Analg.* 2024;138(4):782-793. PMID: 37467164.
2. Al Shabeeb RQ, Lee E, El Shatanofy M, et al. Impact of COVID-19 specific simulation training in improving intubators' level of comfort during intubations of COVID-19 patients - Results from a USA national survey. Trends Anaesth Crit Care. 2022;43:17-22. PMID: 38620697; PMCID: PMC8784652.
3. Putnam EM, Rochlen LR, Alderink E, et al. Virtual reality simulation for critical pediatric airway management training. J Clin Transl Res. 2021;7(1):93-99. Published 2021 Feb 2. PMID: 34104812; PMCID: PMC8177020.

Bougie or stylet in critical care intubation

41

Why this topic is important

Emergency tracheal intubation is a critical intervention in the intensive care unit (ICU) and emergency department. First-attempt success is vital to minimize life-threatening complications, including hypoxemia, hypotension, and cardiac arrest. Two commonly used tools to guide endotracheal tubes during intubation are the bougie and stylet. The choice between these devices can influence outcomes, particularly in patients with difficult airways.

Recent findings from the BOUGIE trial revealed no significant overall difference in first-attempt success between bougie and stylet use in critically ill adults. However, traditional randomized trial methods may not capture individual variability in treatment effects. A secondary analysis by Seitz et al. (2023) applied machine learning techniques to the trial data, identifying patient and operator characteristics that predict individual benefits from each device. These insights could enable personalized intubation strategies, improving outcomes.

Objectives of this update

- Summarize findings from the machine learning analysis comparing bougie and stylet in tracheal intubation.
- Identify characteristics that influence individualized treatment effects.
- Discuss implications for clinical practice and future research.

What is new

- Machine learning revealed significant individualized treatment effects (ITEs) favoring either bougie or stylet based on patient and operator factors.
- Difficult airway characteristics, body mass index (BMI), severity of illness, and operator experience were key predictors of treatment effects.
- Despite no average treatment effect in the trial, the analysis demonstrated that tailoring device choice to individual characteristics could optimize outcomes.

Key findings

Machine learning approach

- Causal forest model: This method analyzed baseline patient and operator characteristics to predict ITEs, identifying which device (bougie or stylet) would maximize each patient's first-attempt success.
- Validation: Predictions were validated in a separate cohort, confirming the model's ability to discriminate treatment effects.

Individualized treatment effects

- Patients with high severity of illness (e.g., elevated Acute Physiology and Chronic Health Evaluation [APACHE] II scores) and higher FiO_2 requirements benefited more from a bougie.
- Patients with difficult airway characteristics (e.g., limited neck mobility, obesity) or higher BMI were likelier to succeed with a stylet.
- Operator experience also influenced outcomes. Clinicians with more bougie intubation experience achieved better results with this device, while less experienced operators performed better with a stylet.

Outcome parameter	Bougie benefit	Stylet benefit
Key patient predictors	Higher APACHE II scores, higher FiO2 requirements, lower Glasgow Coma Scale (GCS) scores	Higher BMI, difficult airway characteristics (e.g., limited neck mobility, obesity)

Clinical outcomes

- Quartiles of benefit: The analysis stratified patients into four groups based on predicted benefits from each device:
    - In the top quartile for bougie benefit, first-attempt success was 90.3% versus 85.1% with a stylet.
    - In the top quartile for stylet benefit, first-attempt success was 81.0% with a stylet versus 60.3% with a bougie.
- Device comparison: While bougie and stylet had no significant difference in overall trial outcomes, the machine learning analysis highlighted substantial variability in individual responses.

Outcome parameter	Bougie benefit	Stylet benefit
First-attempt success rate	90.3%	81.0%

Implications for clinical practice

Personalized device selection

- Tailored strategies: Individualized predictions enable clinicians to choose the most appropriate device for each patient, particularly in challenging airway scenarios.
- Training implications: Emphasizing bougie use during training could improve outcomes for patients who benefit most from this device, particularly in ICUs and emergency departments.

Patient factors

- Difficult airways: Stylet may be preferable for patients with anatomical challenges, such as obesity or limited neck mobility, as it provides rigidity and support during tube advancement.
- Severity of illness: Bougie is better suited for patients requiring rapid oxygenation stabilization due to physiological derangements.

Integration into practice

- Developing clinical decision-support tools based on these findings could assist operators in real-time device selection.
- Incorporating machine learning-based models into electronic health records would facilitate evidence-based, individualized decisions.

Challenges and limitations

Data availability and generalizability

- The BOUGIE trial was conducted in U.S.-based academic centers, which may limit generalizability to other healthcare settings. Further external validation is needed to confirm findings in diverse populations.

Complexity of machine learning models

- While effective, causal forest models can be challenging to interpret, necessitating user-friendly interfaces for clinical implementation.

Need for prospective validation

- The study's findings are hypothesis-generating. Prospective trials are required to evaluate the impact of individualized device selection on clinical outcomes.

Recommendations for future research

- Validation studies: Apply causal forest models in larger, multicenter trials to confirm predictive accuracy across varied patient populations.
- Decision-support development: Create user-friendly tools that integrate predictive models into clinical workflows.
- Operator training: Improve familiarity with both devices to enhance versatility in clinical practice.

Broader implications

The ability to individualize treatment decisions using machine learning represents a significant advancement in critical care. Moving beyond average treatment effects, this approach could optimize outcomes, reduce complications, and improve resource utilization in high-risk procedures like intubation.

The findings also underscore the importance of integrating personalized medicine into routine care, which would allow for more precise and effective interventions in critical settings.

Key takeaways

- ☑ Machine learning identified key predictors of individualized benefits from bougie or stylet during intubation.
- ☑ Difficult airway features favor stylet use, while physiologically compromised patients benefit from a bougie.
- ☑ Personalized device selection based on patient and operator characteristics can enhance first-attempt success rates.
- ☑ Future work should validate these findings and develop clinical decision-support tools for widespread implementation.

Additional recommended reading:

1. Seitz KP, Spicer AB, Casey JD, et al. Individualized Treatment Effects of Bougie versus Stylet for Tracheal Intubation in Critical Illness. *Am J Respir Crit Care Med.* 2023;207(12):1602-1611. PMID: 36877594; PMCID: PMC10273111.
2. Driver BE, Semler MW, Self WH, et al. Effect of Bougie versus Stylet on Intubation Success. *JAMA.* 2021;326:2488-2497. PMID: 34879143; PMCID: PMC8655668.
3. Wang R, Lagakos SW, Ware JH, et al. Statistics in Medicine: Reporting of Subgroup Analyses in Clinical Trials. *N Engl J Med.* 2007;357:2189-2194. PMID: 18032770.

Stylet use and first-attempt intubation success

42

Why this topic is important

First-attempt success (FAS) in tracheal intubation is critical for minimizing complications such as hypoxemia, hemodynamic instability, and airway trauma. Achieving FAS is particularly challenging in intensive care units (ICUs), where emergent settings compound anatomical and physiological complexities. Since intubation is one of the most commonly performed procedures in the ICU, often for acute respiratory failure, optimizing techniques to increase FAS is vital for improving patient outcomes.

The STYLETO trial[1], a multicenter randomized controlled study, explored the impact of using a stylet in conjunction with an endotracheal tube compared to using an endotracheal tube alone during intubation. The findings highlight the utility of the stylet as a cost-effective tool for improving FAS while maintaining comparable safety. While the STYLETO trial used direct laryngoscopy as the primary technique, video laryngoscopy is rapidly emerging as the "go-to" method for routine intubations due to its superior visualization and ease of use, particularly in challenging airway scenarios.

Objectives of this update

- Assess the effect of using a stylet on FAS in critically ill adults.
- Explore safety outcomes associated with stylet use during intubation.
- Provide practical recommendations for integrating stylet use into airway management protocols.

What is new

The STYLETO trial demonstrated that:

- The addition of a stylet increased FAS from 71.5% (endotracheal tube alone) to 78.2% (endotracheal tube + stylet), with a statistically significant absolute risk difference of 6.7%.
- Complication rates, including traumatic injuries, were similar between groups.
- The study's pragmatic design reinforces its applicability to real-world ICU settings.
- Emerging evidence supports combining stylet use with video laryngoscopy, further enhancing intubation success rates in patients with anteriorly positioned airways.

Findings from the STYLETO trial

First-attempt intubation success

The primary outcome of FAS was significantly improved with the use of a stylet:

- **Absolute improvement:** 6.7%.
- **The number needed to treat (NNT):** 15, meaning one FAS failure was prevented for every 15 patients intubated using a stylet.
- **Subgroup consistency:** Benefits were observed across most subgroups, including patients with acute respiratory failure, those requiring rapid sequence induction, and patients with moderate to high Mallampati scores.

Safety outcomes

Stylet use did not result in a higher rate of complications:

- **Traumatic injuries:** Comparable rates between stylet (4.0%) and non-stylet (3.6%) groups.
- **Severe complications:** Hypoxemia (SpO_2 < 80%), hemodynamic collapse, and cardiac arrest were similar between groups.
- **Secondary outcomes:** ICU length of stay, ventilator-free days, and mortality rates were unaffected by stylet use.

Practical advantages of stylet use

- **Ease of availability:** Stylets are inexpensive and widely accessible.
- **Operator-independent utility:** Unlike video-laryngoscopy, which requires familiarity and training, stylets can be used effectively by operators with varying experience levels.
- **Compatibility with advanced tools:** Stylets complement videolaryngoscopes, particularly those with hyperangulated blades.

Why first-attempt success matters

Achieving FAS during intubation is essential for reducing patient morbidity:

1. **Minimizes hypoxemia:** Each additional attempt increases the risk of desaturation, particularly in critically ill patients with reduced oxygen reserves.
2. **Reduces airway trauma:** Repeated intubation attempts are associated with higher rates of mucosal injury and bleeding.
3. **Limits hemodynamic instability:** Prolonged or repeated laryngoscopy can exacerbate hypotension and other cardiovascular responses.
4. **Improves efficiency:** Reducing the time required for successful intubation minimizes exposure of healthcare workers to potential pathogens, especially relevant during pandemics like COVID-19.

Implications for clinical practice

Integrating stylet use

The study supports the routine use of a stylet in ICU intubation, particularly for high-risk scenarios:

1. **Patient selection:**
    - Favor stylet use in patients with predicted difficult airways (e.g., high Mallampati scores, restricted neck mobility).
    - Use as a default for rapid sequence induction.
2. **Training and familiarity:**
    - Ensure all ICU staff are proficient in stylet-assisted intubation to maximize its benefits.
    - Incorporate stylet techniques into simulation-based training programs.

Pairing with videolaryngoscopy

- Stylet use synergizes with videolaryngoscopy, improving tube advancement in patients with anteriorly positioned airways.
- Consider combining stylet and VL techniques in patients where direct laryngoscopy might fail.

Revising protocols

Hospitals should update airway management protocols to recommend stylet use for ICU intubations. Protocol revisions should include:

- **Pre-procedure preparation:**
  - Ensure stylets are included in airway carts.
  - Incorporate stylet use into checklist-based preparations.
- **Post-procedure evaluation:**
  - Monitor for complications like mucosal injury to reinforce safety data.

Addressing concerns about stylet use

Injury risks

Critics of stylet use often cite concerns about mucosal trauma or tracheal injury. However, the STYLETO trial demonstrated no significant difference in injury rates between stylet and non-stylet groups. To further mitigate risks:

- Use a bend angle of 25-35° at the stylet's distal tip to facilitate smooth insertion.
- Remove the stylet gently once the tube is past the vocal cords.

Generalizability

While the STYLETO trial focused on ICU settings, its findings likely extend to emergency departments and pre-hospital environments. The low cost and simplicity of stylet use make it a valuable tool in diverse clinical contexts.

Limitations of the STYLETO trial

Although the results are robust, certain limitations should be acknowledged:

1. **Unblinded design:**
   - Operators were aware of group assignments, potentially introducing bias. However, objective outcomes like FAS mitigate this concern.
2. **Setting-specific results:**
   - The trial was conducted in ICUs, limiting direct extrapolation to operating rooms or pre-hospital care.
3. **Focus on FAS:**
   - The study was not powered to detect differences in secondary outcomes like ICU mortality or length of stay.

Key takeaways

☑ Stylet use during intubation significantly increases first-attempt success in critically ill adults, with an absolute improvement of 6.7%.

☑ Complication rates are similar between stylet and non-stylet approaches, reinforcing the safety of stylet use.

☑ Stylets are cost-effective, widely available, and require minimal training, making them an ideal addition to airway management strategies.

☑ Hospitals should incorporate stylet use into airway protocols, emphasizing its role in achieving FAS and reducing the risk of complications.

Additional recommended reading:

1. Jaber S, Rolle A, Godet T, et al. Effect of the use of an endotracheal tube and stylet versus an endotracheal tube alone on first-attempt intubation success: a multicentre, randomised clinical trial. *Intensive Care Med*. 2021;47(6):653-664. PMID: 34032882; PMCID: PMC8144872.

2. Driver BE, Prekker ME, Klein LR, et al. Effect of use of a bougie vs endotracheal tube and stylet on first-attempt intubation success among patients with difficult airways undergoing emergency intubation: a randomized clinical trial. *JAMA*. 2018;319(20):2179-2189. PMID: 29800096; PMCID: PMC6134434.

3. De Jong A, Rolle A, Molinari N, et al. First-attempt success is associated with fewer complications related to intubation in the intensive care unit. *Intensive Care Med*. 2020;46(6):1278-1280. PMID: 32322917.

4. Tollman J, Ahmed Z. Efficacy of tracheal tube introducers and stylets for endotracheal intubation in the prehospital setting: a systematic review and meta-analysis. Eur J Trauma Emerg Surg. 2022;48(3):1723-1735. PMID: 34333690; PMCID: PMC9192420.

Airway safety and risk management

Adverse event risk patterns in airway management

43

Why this topic is important

Airway management is a high-stakes component of anesthesia and critical care, where minor errors can escalate into major complications. The Swiss cheese model of safety posits that adverse events arise from cumulative failures in multiple system layers. By understanding patterns of consecutive adverse events, clinicians can target risk reduction strategies and refine airway management protocols to improve patient safety.

Huber et al. (2023) applied Bayesian network analysis to explore how consecutive airway events evolve and how targeted interventions can break these chains. The study demonstrates the value of this probabilistic approach in quantifying risk and improving outcomes, offering a practical framework for enhancing patient safety and reducing complications.

Objectives of this update

- Highlight patterns of risk progression during airway management, based on Bayesian network analysis.
- Examine the impact of targeted strategies on reducing initial and consecutive airway events.
- Provide practical recommendations for implementing evidence-based interventions in clinical settings.

What is new

The study by Huber et al. introduces a novel application of Bayesian networks to quantify relationships between airway management events:

- Conditional probabilities revealed typical sequences of adverse events, such as difficult bag-mask ventilation (BMV) often preceding Cormack-Lehane grade ≥ 3 views during intubation.
- Targeted airway management strategies reduced the likelihood of initial adverse events but showed limited efficacy in obese patients.
- Improvements in handling tracheal tube-related events increased the probability of no further complications from 43.3% to 56.4% after implementing targeted changes.

Key findings from Bayesian analysis

Baseline risks and sequential patterns

The study analyzed 6,170 adult cases of airway management, recording adverse events in both elective and emergency procedures. Key observations include:

1. **Common initial events:**
   - The most frequent first events were:
     - Difficult BMV: 16.3%.
     - Tracheal tube-related events (e.g., cuff leaks, tube misplacement): 18.7%.
     - Hypoxemia ($SpO_2 < 90\%$): 14.4%.
   - These first events often triggered subsequent complications, emphasizing the importance of successful initial airway management.
2. **Consecutive events:**
   - Patients with one adverse event had a 42.4% chance of experiencing a second, compared to a baseline first-event risk of 17.1%.
   - Common sequences included:
     - Difficult BMV leading to difficult intubation (Cormack-Lehane grade ≥ 3).
     - Tracheal tube-related events necessitating the unplanned use of special equipment.

Patient-specific factors

1. **Obesity:**
   - Patients with a body mass index (BMI) ≥30 kg/m^2 exhibited significantly higher risks of both initial and consecutive events.
   - This group benefited less from the targeted interventions studied, underscoring the complexity of managing obese airways.
2. **ASA physical status:**
   - The incidence of adverse events was higher among patients classified as ASA 3-6, but the interventions showed comparable efficacy across ASA groups, indicating broad applicability.

Targeted interventions and their outcomes

Preoxygenation and apneic oxygenation

- **Rationale:**
  - Preoxygenation maximizes oxygen reserves, reducing the risk of hypoxemia during apnea.
  - Apneic oxygenation through a high-flow nasal cannula or low-flow nasal oxygen extends the safe apnea period.
- **Impact:**
  - Improved oxygenation reduced the incidence of hypoxemia as an initial adverse event and decreased the likelihood of subsequent complications.

Early neuromuscular blockade

- **Rationale:**
  - Neuromuscular blocking agents improve intubation conditions by reducing patient movement, relaxing the vocal cords, and optimizing visualization.
- **Impact:**
  - Early administration of NMB significantly lowered rates of difficult intubation and the need for multiple attempts.

Videolaryngoscopy

- **Rationale:**
  - VL enhances visualization of the glottis, reducing failed intubations and improving first-pass success rates.
- **Impact:**
  - The use of VL after failed initial attempts reduced the risk of esophageal intubation and unplanned equipment use.

Structured protocols and checklists

- **Rationale:**
  - Checklists ensure readiness by verifying equipment availability, patient positioning, and team preparedness.
- **Impact:**
  - Implementation of pre-induction checklists reduced the likelihood of tracheal tube-related events and improved outcomes across diverse patient groups.

Practical recommendations for clinicians

Pre-induction strategies

1. **Comprehensive risk assessment:**
   - Identify predictors of difficult airway management, such as obesity, limited neck mobility, or craniofacial abnormalities, during the preoperative evaluation.
2. **Structured preparation:**
   - Use a pre-induction checklist to confirm readiness, ensuring the availability of videolaryngoscopes, bougies, and rescue devices like supraglottic airway devices (SGAs).

During airway management

1. **Optimize first attempts:**
   - Administer preoxygenation and consider apneic oxygenation to extend the safe apnea time.
   - Limit intubation attempts to two per provider to minimize complications.
   - Escalate to senior personnel or advanced tools (e.g., VL or flexible bronchoscopes) after initial failures.
2. **Early interventions for complications:**
   - Address difficult BMV promptly with SGAs or by adjusting patient positioning (e.g., head-elevated laryngoscopy position).
   - Use suction aggressively to clear the airway of secretions or blood that may impede visualization.

Post-event management

1. **Escalation pathways:**
   - Anticipate potential follow-up complications after an initial event and have strategies ready to address them.
   - For example, verify placement with capnography after a tracheal tube-related event and prepare for backup ventilation options.
2. **Team communication:**
   - Maintain closed-loop communication to ensure clarity and prevent errors during airway management.

Improving outcomes through systems-based approaches

Airway management bundles

Develop institutional bundles incorporating best practices:

- Pre-induction checklists.
- Standardized use of advanced tools like videolaryngoscopy for high-risk cases.
- Clear escalation protocols for difficult airways, emphasizing the early involvement of senior clinicians.

Data-driven quality improvement

Leverage data collection and analysis to monitor outcomes and refine protocols:

- Use tools like Bayesian analysis to identify recurring risk patterns in your institution.
- Track the impact of interventions on adverse event rates and share findings with the team to promote accountability and improvement.

Addressing challenges in specific populations

Managing obesity in airway management

- Obese patients are at higher risk for hypoxemia, difficult BMV, and failed intubations.
- Interventions for this group should include:
    - Ramp positioning to align the external auditory meatus with the sternal notch.
    - Routine use of VL for intubation.
    - Proactive oxygenation strategies, such as HFNO, during induction and extubation.

Improving training for challenging scenarios

- Regular simulation-based training enhances preparedness for managing consecutive events.
- Focus on both technical skills (e.g., VL use) and non-technical skills (e.g., team coordination) to optimize performance in real-world situations.

Key takeaways

☑ Airway management carries inherent risks, with minor events often triggering a cascade of complications.

☑ Bayesian analysis identifies predictable patterns of adverse events, enabling targeted prevention and intervention strategies.

☑ Interventions such as preoxygenation, neuromuscular blockade, videolaryngoscopy, and structured checklists reduce the likelihood of both initial and consecutive events.

☑ Obesity remains a significant challenge, requiring tailored approaches to improve outcomes in this high-risk population.

☑ Incorporating these evidence-based practices into institutional protocols can enhance patient safety and reduce complications.

Additional recommended reading:

1. Huber M, Greif R, Pedersen TH, et al. Risk patterns of consecutive adverse events in airway management: a Bayesian network analysis. *Br J Anaesth*. 2023;130(3):368-378. PMID: 36564247.
2. Pedersen TH, Ueltschi F, Hornshaw T, et al. Optimisation of airway management strategies: a prospective before-and-after study on events related to airway management. *Br J Anaesth*. 2021;127(5):798-806. PMID: 34535275.
3. Groombridge C, Maini A, Olaussen A, et al. Impact of a targeted bundle of audit with tailored education and an intubation checklist to improve airway management in the emergency department. *Emerg Med J*. 2020;37:576-580. PMID: 32554746.

Optimizing airway safety in anesthesia

44

Why this topic is important

Airway management is a critical component of anesthesia practice, and while generally safe, it is associated with significant risks of both minor and major adverse events. Issues such as difficult bag-mask ventilation, hypoxemia, and esophageal intubation can compromise patient safety and lead to severe complications, including perioperative morbidity and mortality.

The study by Pedersen et al. 2021 highlights the importance of a proactive and systematic approach to improving airway safety. By implementing a targeted bundle of strategies, they demonstrated a measurable reduction in airway-related adverse events. These findings emphasize the value of tailored interventions that address anesthesia departments' specific needs and challenges. Importantly, the study underscores that even established practices benefit from continuous evaluation and refinement, particularly as new tools and techniques become available.

Objectives of this update

- Review the impact of tailored interventions on reducing airway-related adverse events during anesthesia.
- Highlight the importance of incorporating checklists, advanced equipment, and enhanced training in airway management practices.
- Provide actionable insights for optimizing patient safety in routine and high-risk cases.

What is new

- Implementing a five-step bundle reduced the incidence of airway-related events from 15.4% to 11.4%.
- Significant improvements were observed in first-attempt success rates for intubation and reductions in hypoxemia and esophageal intubations.
- Increased use of videolaryngoscopy as a primary tool led to better visualization and fewer complications during tracheal intubation.

Key findings

Study overview

This prospective before-and-after study was conducted in a university hospital and included 7,454 patients undergoing anesthesia. Airway-related events were documented during a baseline phase (2015) and after implementing a targeted intervention bundle, followed by a year-long assessment period (2016).

Impact of interventions

1. Reduction in overall events: The proportion of cases with airway-related events dropped significantly from 15.4% at baseline to 11.4% after implementing the intervention bundle, highlighting its overall effectiveness.

2. Improvements in specific outcomes: Difficult bag-mask ventilation decreased from 3.8% to 2.7%, demonstrating the benefit of enhanced preoxygenation techniques and immediate muscle relaxant use in improving ventilation efficiency.

3. Incidence of hypoxemia: Hypoxemia fell from 3.8% to 2.9%, showing that consistent oxygen delivery and apneic oxygenation strategies can prevent oxygen desaturation during critical phases.

4. Esophageal intubation rates: The incidence of esophageal intubation was reduced from 1.3% to 0.8%, reflecting improved glottic visualization and accurate tracheal tube placement with the increased use of videolaryngoscopy.

5. Videolaryngoscopy adoption: The use of video laryngoscopy as the primary intubation tool increased from 3.0% to 9.2%, correlated with better first-attempt success rates and fewer Cormack-Lehane grade 3 or 4 views.

Recommendations for practice

Key elements of the intervention bundle

1. Preoxygenation and apneic oxygenation: Ensure end-tidal oxygen levels reach ≥ 90% before induction by providing adequate preoxygenation and maintaining oxygen delivery during apnea using low-flow nasal oxygen (2-4 L/min) to prevent hypoxemia.
2. Administration of neuromuscular blocking agents: Administer muscle relaxants immediately after the loss of consciousness to improve the efficiency of bag-mask ventilation and facilitate smoother intubation attempts.
3. Checklists for safety and communication: Implement a pre-induction airway-safety checklist to confirm equipment readiness, assign team roles, and establish a clear backup plan to address unexpected difficulties.
4. Handover to senior staff after failed attempts: After two unsuccessful intubation attempts, ensure airway management responsibility is transferred to the most experienced team member to optimize success and prevent complications.
5. Videolaryngoscopy as a primary tool: Encourage the routine use of videolaryngoscopes for intubation, as this tool provides superior glottic visualization, improves first-attempt success rates, and reduces the risk of adverse events.

Broader implications

The results of this study underscore the importance of continuous quality improvement in airway management. Targeted interventions, when tailored to a department's specific challenges, can significantly enhance patient safety. The incorporation of video laryngoscopy and structured team communication has proven particularly effective in reducing errors and complications.

These findings pave the way for similar studies in other institutions to determine the generalizability of these interventions. Additionally, multicenter trials could help refine these strategies and establish standardized guidelines for airway management in anesthesia. Emphasizing team-based education and regular practice of airway management scenarios will ensure that these improvements are sustained and scalable across healthcare systems.

Key takeaways

- ☑ Targeted interventions reduced airway-related events from 15.4% to 11.4%.
- ☑ Significant reductions were observed in hypoxemia, difficult bag-mask ventilation, and esophageal intubations.
- ☑ Videolaryngoscopy enhanced glottic visualization and intubation success.
- ☑ Pre-induction checklists and structured communication minimized errors.
- ☑ Ongoing training and adoption of advanced tools are essential for sustaining improvements.

Additional recommended reading:

1. Pedersen TH, Ueltschi F, Hornshaw T, et al. Optimisation of airway management strategies: A prospective before-and-after study on events related to airway management. *Br J Anaesth*. 2021;127(5):798-806. PMID: 34535275.
2. Cook TM, Woodall N, Harper J, et al. Major complications of airway management in the UK: Results of the fourth national audit project. *Br J Anaesth*. 2011;106(5):617-631. PMID: 21447488.
3. Frerk C, Mitchell VS, McNarry AF, et al. Difficult Airway Society 2015 guidelines for management of unanticipated difficult intubation in adults. *Br J Anaesth*. 2015;115(6):827-848. PMID: 26556848; PMCID: PMC4650961.

Miscellaneous

Etomidate and ketamine in emergency intubation

45

Why this topic is important

Emergency endotracheal intubation (EEI) is a critical procedure for managing critically ill patients, often performed under high-stakes conditions where optimizing patient outcomes is paramount. Selecting an appropriate induction agent is crucial, as it directly impacts procedural success and patient survival.

Etomidate and ketamine are widely regarded for their hemodynamic stability and rapid onset, making them popular choices for EEI. However, the choice between these agents remains controversial. While etomidate is associated with adrenal suppression, ketamine may increase the risk of post-induction hypotension. This ongoing debate emphasizes the importance of evidence-based guidance to optimize decision-making. The study by Matchett et al. (2022) offers valuable insights into these two agents' comparative efficacy and safety, focusing on survival outcomes and hemodynamic stability.

Objectives of this update

- Summarize the key findings from Matchett et al.'s randomized trial comparing etomidate and ketamine for EEI.
- Highlight the implications of these findings for clinical practice, particularly in managing critically ill patients.
- Provide practical recommendations for using etomidate and ketamine based on patient-specific factors.

What is new

- In critically ill patients, ketamine was associated with higher Day 7 survival rates compared to etomidate (85.1% vs. 77.3%).
- Both agents showed similar Day 28 survival rates, suggesting no long-term survival advantage for ketamine.
- Ketamine was linked to increased post-induction hemodynamic support requirements, raising questions about its impact on cardiovascular stability.

Key findings

Study design and outcomes

The randomized clinical trial included 801 critically ill patients requiring EEI. Participants were randomized to receive either etomidate (0.2-0.3 mg/kg) or ketamine (1-2 mg/kg) as the induction agent. The study's primary endpoint was survival at Day 7, with secondary outcomes including Day 28 survival, ICU length of stay, and post-induction hemodynamic outcomes.

1. Day 7 survival:
   - Ketamine group: 85.1% survival.
   - Etomidate group: 77.3% survival.
   - The hazard ratio for death with etomidate was 1.6.
2. Day 28 survival:
   - No significant differences were observed between the two groups.
3. Hemodynamic stability:
   - Patients receiving ketamine required more frequent vasopressor support post-induction (26.0% vs. 18.8%).
   - Cardiovascular collapse was also more common in the ketamine group (25.1% vs. 17.4%).

Hemodynamic and metabolic considerations

- Etomidate suppresses adrenal cortisol synthesis via 11-beta hydroxylase inhibition, potentially compromising stress responses during critical illness.
- Ketamine's sympathomimetic properties often provide cardiovascular stability, yet this study was associated with greater hemodynamic interventions post-intubation.

Clinical relevance of findings

- Ketamine's early survival benefit on day 7 suggests it may be preferable for patients at high risk of early mortality.
- The absence of significant differences on day 28 raises questions about its long-term impact and reinforces the need for individualized drug selection.

Recommendations for practice

Agent selection based on patient factors

1. Etomidate:
   - Ideal for patients with pre-existing cardiovascular instability or shock, as it minimizes acute hemodynamic perturbations.
   - Use cautiously in patients at risk for adrenal insufficiency or those requiring prolonged mechanical ventilation.
2. Ketamine:
   - Given its bronchodilatory effects, it is preferable for patients with reactive airway disease or bronchospasm.
   - Consider avoiding it in patients with severe cardiovascular compromise due to potential hypotension.

Practical strategies during EEI

- Pre-induction preparation: Ensure adequate preoxygenation and establish vascular access for rapid administration of vasopressors if required.
- Induction dose adjustments: Tailor doses to the patient's hemodynamic profile and clinical condition.
- Post-intubation management: Monitor for hemodynamic instability and promptly address adrenal insufficiency or hypotension.

Broader implications

The findings from this trial underscore the complexity of induction agent selection in EEI. Both etomidate and ketamine have distinct advantages and limitations, necessitating a patient-centered approach. This study highlights the need for continued research into induction agents that balance hemodynamic stability with longer-term survival benefits.

Future directions include:

- Developing predictive models to guide drug selection based on patient-specific risk factors.
- Conducting multicenter trials to validate findings and explore their applicability across diverse patient populations.
- Investigating alternative induction agents or combinations to optimize safety and efficacy in critically ill patients.

Key takeaways

- ☑ In this study, ketamine demonstrated higher Day 7 survival rates compared to etomidate, though no differences were observed at Day 28.
- ☑ While ketamine may improve short-term outcomes, it was associated with increased post-induction vasopressor requirements and cardiovascular collapse.
- ☑ Etomidate remains a reliable choice for hemodynamically fragile patients but carries risks of adrenal suppression.
- ☑ Individualized drug selection and vigilant post-intubation monitoring are essential to improve outcomes in EEI.

Additional recommended reading:

1. Matchett G, Gasanova I, Riccio CA, et al. Etomidate versus ketamine for emergency endotracheal intubation: A randomized clinical trial. *Intensive Care Med.* 2022;48:78-91. PMID: 34904190.
2. Jabre P, Combes X, Lapostolle F, et al. Etomidate versus ketamine for rapid sequence intubation in acutely ill patients: A multicenter randomized trial. *Lancet.* 2009;374:293-300. PMID: 19573904.
3. Mohr NM, Pape SG, Runde D, et al. Etomidate use is associated with less hypotension than ketamine for emergency department sepsis intubations: A NEAR cohort study. *Acad Emerg Med.* 2020;27:1140—1149. PMID: 32602974; PMCID: PMC8711033.

Emergency anaphylaxis management with updated guidelines

46

Why this topic is important

Anaphylaxis is a severe, systemic allergic reaction that can escalate rapidly, leading to life-threatening outcomes if not managed promptly and effectively. It manifests across multiple systems, including respiratory, cardiovascular, and gastrointestinal, often presenting symptoms such as airway obstruction, hypotension, and severe bronchospasm. The incidence of anaphylaxis has been on the rise globally, with studies reporting lifetime prevalence rates between 0.05% and 5.1% in different regions.

Despite its critical nature, anaphylaxis remains underdiagnosed and undertreated, largely due to variability in clinical recognition and delayed intervention. High-quality, evidence-based guidelines are necessary to equip healthcare providers with standardized protocols to mitigate the risks associated with this medical emergency. Recent recommendations emphasize using first-line therapies like epinephrine while addressing the nuances of management in complex scenarios.

Objectives of this update

- Provide a comprehensive overview of the updated clinical practice guidelines for managing anaphylaxis.
- Highlight critical recommendations for diagnosis, medication use, and emergency interventions.
- Discuss strategies for enhancing patient safety and preventing complications in diverse healthcare settings.

What is new

- Adoption of a four-tier grading system for classifying anaphylaxis severity, aiding in tailored interventions.
- Expanded evidence supporting intramuscular (IM) epinephrine as the gold standard for first-line treatment.
- Emphasis on post-treatment monitoring and patient education to reduce recurrence and improve outcomes.

Key findings

Diagnosis and classification of anaphylaxis

Updated guidelines recommend using the American National Institute of Allergy and Infectious Diseases/Food Allergy and Anaphylaxis Network (NIAID/FAAN) diagnostic criteria to ensure early and accurate identification of anaphylaxis. These criteria emphasize the presence of acute onset symptoms involving at least two organ systems, including skin, respiratory, cardiovascular, or gastrointestinal systems. The guidelines also advocate for grading severity from I (mild) to IV (cardiorespiratory arrest), helping clinicians determine the urgency and intensity of treatment.

Epinephrine as the cornerstone of treatment

Epinephrine remains the first-line treatment for anaphylaxis, recommended for all patients classified as Grade II or higher. Key points include:

- Route and dose: IM injection into the mid-anterolateral thigh is preferred due to its rapid absorption and efficacy. The recommended dose is 0.01 mg/kg (maximum 0.5 mg for adults and 0.3 mg for children), repeatable every 5-15 minutes as needed.

- IV administration: Reserved for severe cases (Grade IV) or situations where IM epinephrine is ineffective, requiring careful monitoring to avoid complications like arrhythmias and hypertension.

- Safety: There are no absolute contraindications for epinephrine in life-threatening anaphylaxis. Caution is advised in elderly patients or those with cardiovascular conditions, but the benefits of timely administration outweigh the potential risks.

Supportive and second-line treatments

- H1 antagonists relieve skin and mucosal symptoms but are only recommended after epinephrine. Their role in mitigating biphasic reactions remains uncertain.

- Glucocorticoids: While evidence supporting their efficacy in preventing prolonged or recurrent symptoms is weak, they are often administered to manage bronchospasm or prevent biphasic anaphylaxis.

- Inhaled β2 agonists are effective in alleviating bronchospasm and wheezing, particularly in patients with respiratory involvement.

Airway management

Severe anaphylaxis with airway compromise necessitates prompt action:

- Endotracheal intubation: Recommended in cases of respiratory failure or significant airway edema.

- Cricothyroidotomy: Considered a last-resort measure in "cannot intubate, cannot oxygenate" scenarios, especially in patients with complete upper airway obstruction.

Post-emergency care and prevention

- Patients should be monitored for at least 12 hours after stabilization, as biphasic anaphylaxis can occur within this period. Vital signs, urine output, and oxygen saturation should be continuously assessed.

- Comprehensive patient education on allergen avoidance, using epinephrine auto-injectors, and recognizing early symptoms of anaphylaxis is crucial to prevent recurrence. Healthcare providers should also document and report drug-induced anaphylaxis to improve future care protocols.

Recommendations for practice

During anaphylaxis

1. Administer IM epinephrine immediately at the first suspicion of anaphylaxis (Grade II or higher). Do not delay treatment while awaiting diagnostic confirmation.

2. Ensure continuous monitoring of cardiovascular and respiratory functions, particularly when IV epinephrine or other medications are used.

Post-treatment and discharge

1. Observe patients for 12-24 hours post-treatment to detect late-phase or biphasic reactions.
2. Equip patients with epinephrine auto-injectors and provide training on their use.
3. Encourage follow-up with allergists or immunologists for comprehensive evaluation and long-term management plans.

Anaphylaxis Management: Recognize, Act, Monitor	
1. Recognition	Symptoms involving ≥ 2 organ systems (e.g., skin, respiratory, cardiovascular, gastrointestinal).
2. Grading severity	Use a color-coded 4-tier system (I-IV).
3. Immediate action	Administer IM epinephrine (0.01 mg/kg, mid-anterolateral thigh)
4. Supportive treatments	H1 antagonists, glucocorticoids, and β2 agonists.
5. Airway management	Intubation/cricothyroidotomy (when indicated).
6. Post-emergency monitoring	Minimum 12 hours for biphasic reactions.
7. Education	Auto-injector use, allergen avoidance, follow-up care.

Broader implications

The updated guidelines underscore the critical importance of early recognition and intervention in anaphylaxis. Standardizing diagnostic criteria and emphasizing epinephrine as the first-line treatment can reduce mortality and morbidity significantly. These guidelines apply to emergency departments and are essential for outpatient clinics, perioperative care, and school-based healthcare settings.

Future directions include:

- Enhancing training for healthcare providers on anaphylaxis recognition and treatment.
- Increasing accessibility to epinephrine, particularly in resource-limited settings.
- Conduct research to validate newer therapies and improve management strategies.

Key takeaways

☑ Early administration of IM epinephrine is lifesaving and should never be delayed in suspected anaphylaxis.

☑ The NIAID/FAAN criteria and the four-tier grading system improve diagnostic accuracy and guide tailored interventions.

☑ Comprehensive post-treatment monitoring and patient education are vital to reducing recurrence and ensuring long-term safety.

☑ Collaboration among healthcare providers, patients, and caregivers is crucial for effective management and prevention of anaphylaxis.

Additional recommended reading:

1. Li X, Ma Q, Yin J, et al. A clinical practice guideline for the emergency management of anaphylaxis. *Front Pharmacol.* 2022;13:845689. PMID: 35418863; PMCID: PMC8996305.

2. Muraro A, Worm M, Alviani C, et al. EAACI guidelines: Anaphylaxis (2021 update). Allergy. 2022;77(2):357-377. PMID: 34343358.

3. Pumphrey RSH. Lessons for management of anaphylaxis from a study of fatal reactions. *Clin Exp Allergy.* 2000;30(8):1144-1150. PMID: 10931122.

Pulse oximetry in diagnosing and managing acute respiratory distress syndrome

47

Why this topic is important

Acute respiratory distress syndrome (ARDS) is a life-threatening condition requiring timely diagnosis and intervention. The standard diagnostic approach relies on arterial blood gas analysis to determine the partial pressure of arterial oxygen (PaO_2) relative to the fraction of inspired oxygen (FiO_2). However, this method is invasive, costly, and often inaccessible in resource-limited settings.

Pulse oximetry, by contrast, is non-invasive, readily available, and widely used in clinical settings to monitor oxygen saturation (SpO_2). Recent studies suggest that pulse oximetry-based indices like the SpO_2/FiO_2 ratio could be practical alternatives to PaO_2/FiO_2 for diagnosing ARDS. Leveraging pulse oximetry could expand access to ARDS diagnosis, enhance early recognition, and support global epidemiological studies, particularly in under-resourced environments.

Objectives of this update

- Explain the role of pulse oximetry in ARDS diagnosis and management.
- Compare SpO_2/FiO_2 to PaO_2/FiO_2 for assessing hypoxemia severity.
- Discuss the advantages and limitations of pulse oximetry in ARDS care.
- Highlight its potential in global healthcare and clinical trials.

What is new

- Pulse oximetry-based indices are gaining acceptance as diagnostic and prognostic tools in ARDS.
- The SpO_2/FiO_2 ratio is validated for diagnosing ARDS in settings without arterial blood gas analysis, such as low-resource environments.
- Noninvasive alternatives, such as the respiratory rate and oxygenation (ROX) index and oxygen saturation index (OSI), are increasingly being used for risk stratification and clinical trials.

Key findings

Diagnostic potential of pulse oximetry

- SpO_2/FiO_2 ratio: Proposed as a surrogate for the PaO_2/FiO_2 ratio, the SpO_2/FiO_2 ratio has been validated in multiple studies. A threshold of 315 corresponds to mild ARDS ($PaO_2/FiO_2 \leq 300$ mm Hg), while 235 aligns with moderate-to-severe ARDS ($PaO_2/FiO_2 \leq 200$ mm Hg).
- Resource-limited settings: The Kigali modification of ARDS diagnostic criteria incorporates the SpO_2/FiO_2 ratio, enabling diagnosis in environments without access to arterial blood gas analysis.

Advantages over traditional methods

- Accessibility: Pulse oximetry is available in most healthcare settings, making it a practical alternative in resource-limited areas.
- Continuous monitoring: Unlike intermittent arterial blood gas sampling, pulse oximetry provides real-time data, aiding early detection and intervention.
- Risk-free: Non-invasive and free from complications like iatrogenic anemia or vascular injury associated with frequent arterial sampling.

Emerging tools and indices

- Oxygen saturation index (OSI): This index incorporates mean airway pressure into calculations, providing a more nuanced measure of oxygenation and respiratory failure severity.
- ROX index: Used to predict outcomes in patients on high-flow nasal oxygen (HFNO), this ratio of SpO_2/FiO_2 to respiratory rate identifies patients at high risk of progression to invasive ventilation.

Limitations and challenges

Accuracy considerations

- Perfusion states: Reduced accuracy in patients with poor perfusion or severe hypoxemia.
- Skin pigmentation: Studies suggest potential overestimation of oxygen saturation in individuals with darker skin tones, warranting further investigation.
- Flat dissociation curve: Above SpO_2 values of 97%, pulse oximetry becomes less sensitive to changes in PaO_2, limiting its utility at high oxygen saturation levels.

Diagnostic misclassification

- Relying solely on SpO_2/FiO_2 may result in misclassification of ARDS severity, although the impact on clinical outcomes is minimal compared to the benefits of early recognition.

Implementation hurdles

- Adoption of pulse oximetry-based metrics in ARDS diagnostic criteria would require global consensus and education to ensure accurate use.
- Further validation of non-linear or log-linear imputation methods for estimating PaO_2 from SpO_2 is needed for widespread application.

Strategies for optimization

Research and validation

- **Clinical trials:** To further establish pulse oximetry indices' reliability, include them as inclusion criteria or endpoints in ARDS studies.
- **Population studies:** Investigate the performance of SpO_2/FiO_2 and related indices across diverse patient demographics and settings.

Education and training

- Teach clinicians to interpret pulse oximetry data accurately, particularly its limitations at high saturation levels and in certain patient populations.
- Guide when arterial blood gas analysis is necessary to confirm diagnoses or resolve diagnostic ambiguity.

Resource equity

- Promote the widespread availability of pulse oximeters in resource-limited settings to enhance ARDS diagnosis and management.
- Develop affordable and robust devices tailored for low-income regions.

Broader implications for global health

Adopting pulse oximetry-based metrics could transform ARDS care worldwide by addressing the persistent underdiagnosis of this condition. This approach enables early recognition and management in resource-limited settings, improving patient outcomes. Additionally, pulse oximetry facilitates large-scale epidemiological studies and clinical trials, contributing to a deeper understanding of ARDS.

As global healthcare systems adapt to increasing demands, pulse oximetry is invaluable for enhancing diagnostic accuracy and access. Its integration into ARDS diagnostic frameworks offers a unique opportunity to improve care across diverse settings, fostering equity in critical care medicine.

Key takeaways

☑ Pulse oximetry-based indices like SpO_2/FiO_2 are practical alternatives to PaO_2/FiO_2 for ARDS diagnosis.

☑ These tools are particularly valuable in resource-limited settings, where arterial blood gas analysis may be unavailable.

☑ Emerging indices such as OSI and ROX expand the utility of pulse oximetry in risk stratification and management.

☑ Challenges include reduced accuracy in specific populations and the need for broader validation.

☑ Widespread adoption of pulse oximetry in ARDS care can improve early detection, support global research, and enhance healthcare equity.

Additional recommended reading:

1. Wick KD, Matthay MA, Ware LB. Pulse oximetry for the diagnosis and management of acute respiratory distress syndrome. *Lancet Respir Med*. 2022;10(11):1086-1098. PMID: 36049490; PMCID: PMC9423770.
2. Rice TW, Wheeler AP, Bernard GR, et al. Comparison of the SpO_2/FiO_2 ratio and the PaO_2/FiO_2 ratio in patients with acute lung injury or ARDS. *Chest*. 2007;132:410-417. PMID: 17573487.
3. Roca O, Messika J, Caralt B, et al. Predicting success of high-flow nasal cannula in pneumonia patients with hypoxaemic respiratory failure: the utility of the ROX index. *J Crit Care*. 2016;35:200-205. PMID: 27481760.

Skin pigmentation and pulse oximetry accuracy

48

Why this topic is important

Pulse oximetry is a cornerstone of non-invasive monitoring in clinical practice, especially during the COVID-19 pandemic, where its role in assessing oxygen saturation (SpO_2) became crucial for triaging patients and managing care remotely. This technology, reliant on photoplethysmography (PPG), uses light absorption properties to measure blood oxygen levels. However, growing evidence suggests that pulse oximeters may produce inaccurate readings in individuals with darker skin pigmentation, especially under hypoxic conditions.

Such discrepancies can lead to "occult hypoxemia," where a patient's true arterial oxygen saturation (SaO_2) is dangerously low despite normal SpO_2 readings. Occult hypoxemia is a significant clinical concern, as delayed intervention increases risks of adverse outcomes, including organ failure and death. Addressing these disparities is essential for equitable healthcare delivery and improving device performance across diverse populations.

Objectives of this update

- To assess how skin pigmentation affects the accuracy of pulse oximeters in measuring oxygen saturation.
- To highlight key findings from systematic reviews and bibliometric analyses on this topic.
- To discuss the clinical implications of device inaccuracies and propose recommendations for improving pulse oximeter reliability.

Key findings

A systematic review by Cabanas et al. 2022 examined 41 studies spanning 1976-2022 to explore the relationship between skin pigmentation and pulse oximetry accuracy. Key findings include:

1. Overestimation of SpO_2 in dark-skinned individuals:
   - Most studies identified significant in-accuracies, particularly at low saturation levels, with a consistent trend toward overestimated SpO_2 values in individuals with darker pigmentation.
2. Increased risk of occult hypoxemia:
   - Patients with darker skin were 3 times more likely to experience occult hypoxemia (SaO_2 < 88% with normal SpO_2 readings).
3. Limitations in device calibration:
   - Many pulse oximeters are calibrated using light-skinned populations, leading to errors in populations with darker pigmentation due to the higher melanin content interfering with light absorption.
4. Variability in methods and scales:
   - Studies used different methods to assess skin pigmentation, ranging from subjective descriptions (e.g., "light" or "dark") to objective scales like the Fitzpatrick phototype, contributing to inconsistencies in findings.

Advantages and limitations of pulse oximetry

Strengths:

1. Non-invasive and easy to use:
   - Pulse oximeters provide real-time SpO_2 measurements without invasive procedures like arterial blood gas sampling.
2. Accessibility:
   - Pulse oximetry is a low-cost solution for oxygen saturation monitoring widely used in hospitals, clinics, and homes.

Limitations:

1. Inaccuracy in darker-skinned populations:
   - Melanin in darker skin absorbs light wavelengths used by pulse oximeters, causing SpO_2 readings to overestimate true oxygen saturation.
2. Performance under hypoxic conditions:
   - Device errors are more pronounced when oxygen saturation is low, a critical time for clinical decision-making.
3. Limited generalizability:
   - Current calibration algorithms often need to account for diverse skin pigmentation, leading to disparities in accuracy.

Clinical implications

1. Impact on COVID-19 care:
   - During the pandemic, pulse oximeters were integral to remote monitoring, particularly for identifying silent hypoxia. Inaccurate readings in darker-skinned individuals may have delayed hospitalization or supplemental oxygen administration, contributing to worse outcomes.
2. Implications for critical care:
   - In intensive care settings, inaccurate SpO_2 measurements may affect decisions regarding ventilator management or oxygen therapy, risking both over- and under-treatment.
3. Equity in healthcare:
   - Addressing these disparities is essential to ensure equitable care and improve outcomes for underserved populations.

Recommendations for improving accuracy

1. Standardize calibration processes:
    - Manufacturers should calibrate pulse oximeters using diverse populations to improve performance across all skin tones.
2. Adopt objective skin classification methods:
    - Using standardized scales like the Fitzpatrick phototype instead of subjective descriptions can improve study consistency and device reliability.
3. Educate clinicians:
    - Raise awareness about pulse oximetry's limitations in darker-skinned individuals and encourage the complementary use of arterial blood gas analysis in critical cases.
4. Develop new technologies:
    - Invest in advanced sensors, such as multi-wavelength pulse oximeters, which reduce bias from melanin interference and improve accuracy in diverse populations.

Challenges and future directions

1. Heterogeneity in existing research:
    - Variability in study design, pigmentation classification, and device models complicates the interpretation of results. Future studies should use uniform metho-dologies to ensure robust comparisons.
2. Limited testing under hypoxia:
    - Few studies simulate hypoxic conditions across diverse populations, leaving gaps in understanding device performance during critical clinical scenarios.
3. Resource constraints:
    - High costs of developing and implementing new technologies may limit accessibility in low-resource settings.

Key takeaways

☑ Pulse oximeters overestimate oxygen saturation in darker-skinned individuals, increasing the risk of occult hypoxemia, especially under hypoxic conditions.

☑ Device calibration often excludes diverse skin tones, contributing to disparities in healthcare outcomes.

☑ Objective classification methods and diverse calibration datasets are essential to improving accuracy and equity.

☑ Clinicians should remain vigilant about device limitations and consider alternative methods like arterial blood gas analysis for critical decisions.

Additional recommended reading:

1. Cabanas AM, Fuentes-Guajardo M, Latorre K, et al. Skin Pigmentation Influence on Pulse Oximetry Accuracy: A Systematic Review and Bibliometric Analysis. *Sensors*. 2022;22(9):3402. PMID: 35591092; PMCID: PMC9102088.
2. Feiner JR, Severinghaus JW, Bickler PE. Dark skin decreases the accuracy of pulse oximeters at low oxygen saturation: The effects of oximeter probe type and gender. *Anesth Analg*. 2007;105(6):S18-23. PMID: 18048893.
3. Sjoding MW, Dickson RP, Iwashyna TJ, et al. Racial bias in pulse oximetry measurement. *N Engl J Med*. 2020;383(25):2477-2478. PMID: 33326721; PMCID: PMC7808260

Made in the USA
Las Vegas, NV
30 December 2025

0ff8f7a5-d503-4af2-b0b4-46768e9e6461R02